50% OFF

Online WCC Prep Course!

Dear Customer,

Thank you for your purchase of this WCC Study Guide. Included with your purchase is **discounted access to our online Wound Care Certification Prep Course**. Many WCC courses are needlessly expensive and don't deliver enough value. Our course provides the best WCC prep material, and with discounted access, **you only pay half price**.

We have structured our online course to perfectly complement your printed study guide. The Wound Care Certification Prep Course contains **in-depth lessons** that cover all the most important topics, **550 practice questions** to ensure you feel prepared, and more than **320 digital flashcards**, so you can study while you're on the go.

Online Wound Care Certification Prep Course

Topics Included:

- Assessment
  - Assess Wound Etiology and Status
- Treatment
  - Wound Cleansing
- Re-Evaluation
  - Patient Adherence
- Education
  - Self-Management
- Administration
  - Evidence Based Protocols
- Legal
  - Documentation
- Risk and Prevention
  - Infection Control

Course Features:

- WCC Study Guide
  - Get content that complements our best-selling study guide.
- Full-Length Practice Tests
  - With 550 practice questions, you can test yourself again and again.
- Mobile Friendly
  - If you need to study on the go, the course is easily accessible from your mobile device.
- WCC Flashcards
  - Our course includes a flashcard mode with over 320 content cards to help you study.

To lock in your discounted access, visit mometrix.com/university/wcc or simply scan this QR code with your smartphone. At the checkout page, enter the discount code: **wcc50off**

If you have any questions or concerns, please contact us at support@mometrix.com.

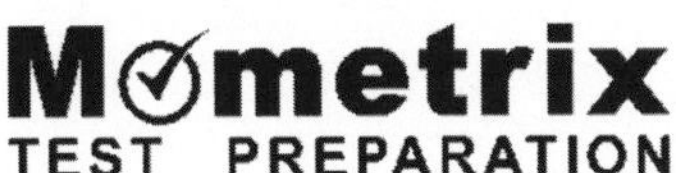

WCC®

Exam Practice Questions

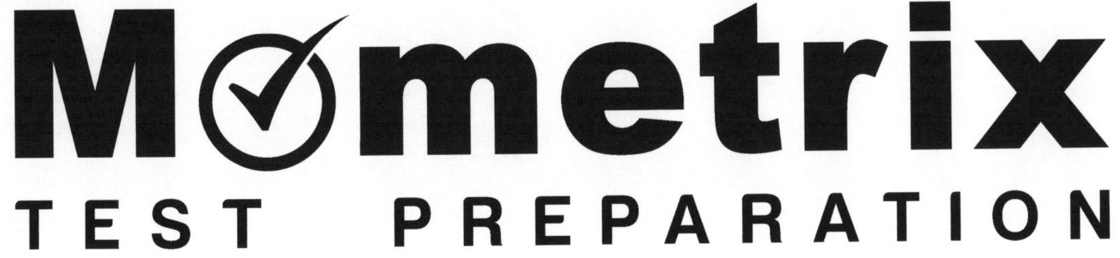

Dear Future Exam Success Story

First of all, **THANK YOU** for purchasing Mometrix study materials!

Second, congratulations! You are one of the few determined test-takers who are committed to doing whatever it takes to excel on your exam. **You have come to the right place.** We developed these practice tests with one goal in mind: to deliver you the best possible approximation of the questions you will see on test day.

Standardized testing is one of the biggest obstacles on your road to success, which only increases the importance of doing well in the high-pressure, high-stakes environment of test day. Your results on this test could have a significant impact on your future, and these practice tests will give you the repetitions you need to build your familiarity and confidence with the test content and format to help you achieve your full potential on test day.

Your success is our success

We would love to hear from you! If you would like to share the story of your exam success or if you have any questions or comments in regard to our products, please contact us at **800-673-8175** or **support@mometrix.com**.

Thanks again for your business and we wish you continued success!

Sincerely,
The Mometrix Test Preparation Team

Written and edited by the Mometrix Exam Secrets Test Prep Team
Printed in the United States of America

TABLE OF CONTENTS

Practice Test #1

1. Which of the following are the three wound factors that most often lead to social isolation?

a. Pain, malodor, and impaired mobility
b. Pain, drainage, and infection
c. Infection, size of wound, and malodor
d. Malodor, drainage, and visible wound

2. A patient with peripheral arterial disease develops an ulcer on the foot. Which of the following is indicated to help determine if the ulcer resulted from ischemia or pressure?

a. Documentation regarding positioning and pressure reduction
b. Assessment of wound character
c. Vascular laboratory/imaging studies
d. Assessment of wound location

3. If a 65-year-old patient's zinc level is 60 mcg/dL, the anticipated effect on the patient's wound is:

a. No effect
b. Accelerated healing
c. Impaired circulation
d. Delayed healing

4. Ultrasound is used in wound care to:

a. Stimulate healing and debride wounds.
b. Decrease bacterial flora.
c. Relax muscles and decrease pain.
d. Increase the tissue temperature.

5. A basic principle of wound care with occlusive dressings is to keep the wound:

a. Cool and dry
b. Warm and dry
c. Warm and moist
d. Cool and moist

6. The best candidate for hyperbaric oxygen therapy is a patient with:

a. Chronic venous ulcers, refractory to standard treatment
b. Chronic diabetic ulcers (Wagner III classification), refractory to standard treatment
c. Newly diagnosed osteomyelitis, recently started on standard treatment
d. Acute wound from trauma to lower leg

7. Which of the following is the best debridement choice for an infected diabetic ulcer with hard gray callus formation at wound edges?

a. Sharp debridement with saucerization or callus removal
b. Autolytic debridement with hydrogels or hydrocolloids
c. Autolytic debridement with transparent film dressing
d. Enzymatic debridement

8. When using the pinch test as an initial assessment of skin turgor and dehydration, which site provides the most accurate results?

a. Skin on top of hand or palm
b. Skin on forehead or sternum
c. Skin on abdomen
d. Skin on forearm or upper arm

9. According to the Modified Wagner Foot Ulcer Classification System, a full-thickness ulcer that extends to the tendon or joint but without abscess or osteomyelitis is classified as:

a. Grade 1
b. Grade 2
c. Grade 3
d. Grade 4

10. When using transparent film dressing for autolytic debridement, how often should dressing changes be scheduled?

a. 8–10 days
b. 5–7 days
c. 3–5 days
d. 1–2 days

11. A chronic ulcer resulting from peripheral vascular insufficiency may remain in which phase of healing for prolonged periods?

a. Hemostasis
b. Inflammation
c. Proliferation
d. Remodeling

12. Hypertrophic scars are most likely to occur:

a. Over joints
b. In dark-skinned patients
c. On the deltoids and earlobes
d. On the upper back and chest

13. When developing a plan of care for a patient who must learn wound management, which of the following would be an appropriate listing of a behavioral outcome?

a. Understands the need to do daily dressing change
b. Accepts mobility limitations
c. Feels that he can manage wound care independently within a few days
d. Able to demonstrate dressing change in 3 days

14. A 15-year-old patient was attacked by a dog and has severe contaminated bite wounds on the legs. The wound will likely be debrided, and closure will likely take place through:

a. Primary healing
b. Secondary healing
c. Tertiary healing
d. Quaternary healing

15. The most common cause of venous outflow obstruction and venous ulceration is:

a. Deep vein thrombosis
b. Trauma
c. Congestive heart failure
d. Obesity

16. When applying an Unna boot for a non-healing venous stasis ulcer, to what tension should the outer self-adhering elastic bandage (Coban) be stretched?

a. 100%
b. 50%
c. 25%
d. 10%

17. Which is the best choice for a support surface for a patient with large stage III and stage IV pressure injuries on multiple turning sites?

a. Alternating air mattress
b. Static flotation (air)
c. Foam
d. Low air loss therapy device

18. A large open wound on the patient's leg is contaminated with dirt, gravel, and other debris. The best approach to cleansing is:

a. Pulsatile lavage only
b. Sharp debridement and pulsatile lavage
c. Hand debridement, large volume irrigation, and pulsatile lavage
d. Large volume irrigation and hand debridement

19. The presence of necrotic tissue and debris that prevent epithelization from occurring is:

a. Bioburden
b. Contamination
c. Colonization
d. Critical colonization

20. Which of the following is the correct documentation of undermining?

a. "Extends 1.8 cm width about one-quarter of wound perimeter."
b. "Extends ¾ inch width by the right lower quadrant of the wound."
c. "Extends 1.8 cm width from 1 o'clock to 4 o'clock."
d. "Extends ¾ inch width from 1 o'clock to 4 o'clock."

21. Patients with a fluidized air/high-air-loss support surface must be carefully monitored for:

a. Bottoming
b. Dehydration
c. Fungal infection
d. Tissue maceration

22. A wound is covered with dry black eschar and is to be debrided with an enzyme. The first step is to:

a. Cover the wound with a layer of enzyme.
b. Thoroughly dry the wound.
c. Crosshatch through the outer layers of the eschar.
d. Do a sharp debridement of the outer layers of the eschar.

23. The healthcare provider is using the ankle-brachial index to assess peripheral arterial disease in a patient. The patient's ankle systolic pressure is 90 mmHg, and their brachial systolic pressure is 120 mmHg for an ABI score of 0.75. This score indicates:

a. Normal reading, asymptomatic
b. Pain, even at rest, limb threatening
c. Critical limb threatening
d. Severe disease, ischemia

24. Painless open ulcers on the pressure points on the bottom of the foot surrounded by calloused skin usually indicate:

a. Arterial insufficiency
b. Neuropathy
c. Chronic venous insufficiency
d. Malignancy

25. Which functional assessment tool measures the 8 activities necessary for an adult to function independently?

a. Barthel Index of Daily Living
b. Instrumental Activities of Daily Living (IADL)
c. Index of Independence of Activities of Daily Living (Katz Index)
d. Palliative Performance Scale

26. If a patient in a hospital that is part of the in-patient prospective payment system has a stage 3 pressure injury present on admission, but this was neither identified nor documented, the hospital:

a. Can amend to documentation at a later date
b. Will receive reimbursement for treatment at a lower rate
c. Cannot claim payment for the pressure injury as a primary or secondary diagnosis
d. Can claim payment for the pressure injury as only a secondary diagnosis

27. The nurse places her hand under a 1.5-inch foam overlay and finds that the overlay has compressed to 0.75 inch, indicating:

a. Bottoming out
b. Adequate support
c. Excess wear
d. Moisture retention

28. Which dietary modification is most important to promote healing for a 50-year-old overweight male who has a third degree burn on his left arm that has had wound debridement and skin grafting?

a. Decreased fats
b. Increased protein
c. Increased carbohydrate
d. Decreased calories

29. Which of the following is an example of a condition/situation that is covered by the CMS surgical dressing benefit?

a. First-degree burn
b. Stage 2 pressure injury
c. Venipuncture site
d. Skin tear

30. Which type of healing would be used for a wound with full-thickness skin loss with wound margins that cannot be approximated and with non-viable wound edges?

a. Superficial wound healing
b. Primary intention
c. Delayed primary intention
d. Secondary intention

31. If a patient's prealbumin level was 16 mg/dL on admission but current testing shows a level of 10 mg/dL, what does this suggest?

a. Indication of acute inadequate protein intake
b. Indication of chronic inadequate protein intake
c. Level within normal limits
d. Indication of infectious process

32. A patient who is receiving oral iron because of an iron deficiency should also be prescribed:

a. Vitamin A
b. Vitamin C
c. Folate
d. Vitamin D

33. What is the NPIAP staging of a pressure injury that is 6 cm in circumference at the surface, but the base is covered with slough and hard dry brown-black eschar?

a. Stage II
b. Stage III
c. Stage IV
d. Unstageable

34. When irrigating a wound, what wound irrigation pressure is needed to effectively cleanse the wound while avoiding trauma?

a. <4 psi
b. 20–30 psi
c. 10–15 psi
d. >15 psi

35. Which type of precautions require that the nurse assistant wear a mask while caring for the patient, that the patient be separated from other patients by at least 3 feet with a curtain separating them, and that the patient be masked during transport to reduce risk of transmission?

a. Standard
b. Contact
c. Airborne
d. Droplet

36. A patient with Charcot arthropathy who has had 2 weeks of compression to reduce edema and inflammation will probably next need a:

a. Total contact cast
b. Half shoe
c. Removable cast walker
d. Foam dressings for cushioning

37. Which of the following is the most effective to prevent pressure injuries on the heels?

a. Foam heel pads
b. Heel dressings
c. Heel elevation device
d. Sheepskin heel pads

38. Which is the best way to move a patient up in bed in order to prevent shear?

a. Place hands under patient's axillary region and pull toward the head of the bed.
b. Ask patient to use trapeze to pull himself/herself up in bed.
c. Use a lift/turning sheet to move patient toward the head of the bed.
d. Lower the head of the bed and elevate the knees and ask patient to slide upward.

39. The initial treatment to relieve the itching and prevent excoriation resulting from venous dermatitis is:

a. Topical antihistamine
b. Compression therapy
c. Topical steroids
d. Topical antibiotics

40. Which of the following topical treatments is usually the best choice to reduce infection and odor in a fungating necrotic neoplastic lesion?

a. Dakin's solution
b. Yogurt
c. Hydrogen peroxide
d. Metronidazole

41. The primary problem with using the troughing technique to manage a posterior small bowel fistula in an open abdominal wound is:

a. Adherence
b. Wound contamination
c. Skin excoriation
d. Fungal infection

42. What is the primary implication when assessing a surgical wound on postoperative day 9, the nurse finds no evidence of a healing ridge?

a. Wound is healing slowly.
b. Wound is infected.
c. Wound is at risk of dehiscence or infection.
d. Wound is well healed.

43. What is the primary purpose for applying elbow pads to a patient who exhibits repetitive movement of the arms and legs?

a. To prevent pressure injuries
b. To promote comfort
c. To reduce shear
d. To reduce friction

44. When cleansing a wound in a shower, how far away from the wound should the showerhead be?

a. 2 inches
b. 6 inches
c. 12 inches
d. 24 inches

45. With static compression therapy, how much pressure should high-level compression dressings exert at the ankle?

a. 30–40 mmHg
b. ≤50 mmHg
c. <23 mmHg
d. 10–20 mmHg

46. With Ayello's ASSESSMENTS tool for evaluation of wounds, the "M" refers to:

a. Marginal edges
b. Medications
c. Management
d. Maceration

47. When obtaining a wound culture for anaerobic organisms, what should the healthcare provider do immediately after aspirating exudate from deep within the wound?

a. Squirt the exudate directly into a culture tube.
b. Apply a needle to the syringe and expel all air, then inject the exudate into a culture tube.
c. Apply a needle to the syringe and inject the exudate into a culture tube.
d. Inject the exudate onto a sterile swab and insert that into a culture tube.

48. Which of the following findings on assessment is a risk factor for malnutrition and impaired healing?

a. Weight 95% of ideal body weight for age
b. Wears dentures
c. Drinks 1–2 glasses of wine daily
d. Body Mass Index (BMI) of <18.5

49. Which of the following is an extrinsic factor that may affect wound healing?

a. Wound bioburden
b. Age
c. Nutrition
d. Immunosuppression

50. Which of the following wound types would be the best candidate for negative pressure wound therapy (NPWT)?

a. Second-degree burns on arm
b. Open wound on leg with osteomyelitis
c. Stage III pressure injury with moderate amount of exudate
d. Abdominal wound dehiscence with organs exposed

51. What is the primary advantage of the clock method of measuring a wound as opposed to the greatest length by greatest width (GLBGW) method?

a. GLBGW underestimates wound size and the clock method does not.
b. Clock method is the most commonly used.
c. Clock method requires less precision.
d. Clock method tracks the same site.

52. When testing a diabetic patient's vibratory perception threshold (VPT) with a tuning fork, the healthcare provider should first conduct a preliminary test on the patient's:

a. Lower leg
b. Forehead
c. Forearm
d. Sternum

53. The primary risk factor for development of pressure injuries is:

a. Sensory loss
b. Inactivity
c. Immobility
d. Cognitive impairment

54. When assessing a wound, what is the best way to differentiate between granulation tissue and muscle tissue?

a. Observe for color.
b. Measure temperature difference.
c. Observe for location in wound.
d. Palpate and gently pinch tissue.

55. Which is the best choice for mechanical debridement of a large infected pressure injury on the right hip with undermining and tunneling in a febrile patient who is undergoing cardiac monitoring?

a. Pulsatile lavage with suction
b. Whirlpool
c. Wet-to-dry dressing
d. Flush with 35 mL syringe with size 19 needle

56. The 5 Ps of neurovascular assessment are:

a. Pain, pulselessness, position, paresthesia, paraplegia
b. Pain, pallor, pulselessness, paresthesia, paraplegia
c. Pain, perception, pulselessness, position, paresthesia
d. Pain, pulselessness, perception, pallor, paraplegia

57. When doing a continuous wave Doppler probe assessment of peripheral pulses, the normal phasic flow pattern is:

a. Quadriphasic
b. Triphasic
c. Biphasic
d. Monophasic

58. What is the best debridement choice for a venous ulcer with hard brown adherent eschar covering 60% of the wound?

a. Autolytic with hydrogels
b. Autolytic with transparent film dressing
c. Sharp
d. Enzymatic

59. What does it mean if one week after Apligraf has been applied to a diabetic ulcer, the wound surface appears gelatinous?

a. Infection
b. Rejection
c. Allergic response
d. Normal response

60. According to Krasner's Chronic Wound Pain Experience (CWPE) model, what intervention would be specifically instituted to relieve cyclic acute wound pain?

a. Transcutaneous nerve stimulation
b. Tri-cycle antidepressants
c. Soaking dressing to loosen prior to removal
d. Application of heat

61. Which pressure measurement is indicative of limb ischemia?

a. Ankle pressure <60 mmHg
b. Ankle pressure <40 mmHg
c. Toe pressure <60 mmHg
d. Toe pressure <40 mmHg

62. High compression stockings (50–60 mmHg), class IV, are recommended for:

a. Edema associated with venous insufficiency
b. Edema associated with lymphedema
c. Dependent edema
d. Edema with ulceration

63. What is the best treatment for a patient with peripheral edema whose lower legs are dry, scaly, and pruritic, resulting in slight excoriation from scratching?

a. Warm mineral oil
b. Corticosteroid ointment
c. Domeboro soaks
d. Neosporin

64. What is the primary purpose of applying foam dressing over amorphous hydrogels or alginates for a large pressure injury?

a. Provide protection.
b. Provide cushioning.
c. Prevent adherence to the wound.
d. Remove excess exudate and promote autolysis.

65. Which of the following treatments may be used to reduce hypergranulation in a wound?

a. Povidone iodine
b. Hyaluronic acid (Hyalofill)
c. Hypertonic sodium chloride
d. Silver sulfadiazine

66. Which is the best dressing to apply to protect reddened but intact skin in order to prevent skin breakdown?

a. Foam dressings
b. Hydrocolloids or film dressings
c. Sheet hydrogel
d. Silver dressings

67. When using a lidocaine soak to prevent pain during debridement of an ulcer, how long should the soak be in contact with the wound before beginning debridement?

a. 3–5 minutes
b. 10–15 minutes
c. 20 minutes
d. 30 minutes

68. Pressure dressings to prevent scarring are usually indicated when a wound takes longer than:

a. >7 days to heal
b. >14 days to heal
c. >21 days to heal
d. >28 days to heal

69. When exercising and stretching a scar, maximal stretch is usually indicated by:

a. Onset of pain
b. Reddening of scar
c. Blanching of scar
d. Increase in pain

70. In the acute surgical wound, signs of inflammation are normal for the first:

a. 24 hours
b. 2 days
c. 3 days
d. 4 days

71. A patient with a Braden score of 13 has what chance of developing a pressure injury?

a. No risk (normal finding)
b. Slight risk (50–60%)
c. Moderate risk (65–90%)
d. High risk (90–100%)

72. How many pillows should be placed for pillow bridging to position patients with minimal compression of tissue?

a. 2
b. 3
c. 4
d. 5

73. When assessing venous refill time, venous occlusion is indicated with times of:

a. >3 seconds
b. >10 seconds
c. >20 seconds
d. >30 seconds

74. What intervention is appropriate for a patient with a diabetic ulcer on the great toe, which is swollen, draining, painful, and has purple discoloration?

a. Referral to surgeon
b. Sharp debridement
c. Autolytic debridement
d. Enzymatic debridement

75. The Harris mat is used for:

a. Strengthening exercises
b. Temperature testing to evaluate Charcot's arthropathy
c. Pressure testing for plantar offloading
d. Foot measurements to evaluate swelling

76. Patients with peripheral neuropathy should have professional skin and nail care of the foot:

a. Every 2 weeks
b. Weekly
c. Every 2 months
d. Monthly

77. If 6 months after an artificial hip was implanted the patient develops an infection of the fascia and muscle layers with purulent discharge, the wound would be categorized according to the CDC's Categories of Surgical Wound Infections as:

a. Category 1
b. Category 2
c. Category 3
d. Category 4

78. For the purpose of Medicare reimbursement for home healthcare, which of the following would disqualify a patient from being considered homebound?

a. The patient occasionally attends religious services.
b. The patient works 2 days a week at an office job.
c. The patient walks around the block 2 or 3 times a week.
d. The patient uses a wheelchair to get around.

79. Which of the following data sets is part of essential wound documentation in skilled nursing facilities?

a. Outcomes and Assessment Information Set
b. Health Plan Employers Data and Information Set
c. Uniform Ambulatory Care Data Set
d. Minimum Data Set

80. What transcutaneous oxygen (tcPO2) level indicates that a wound will probably not heal?

a. <20 mmHg
b. <25 mmHg
c. <30 mmHg
d. <35 mmHg

81. According to the NPIAP consensus statement, which of the following patient circumstances may result in unavoidable pressure injuries?

a. Impaired cognitive status
b. Hemodynamic instability that prevents repositioning
c. Peripheral neuropathy that decreases sensation
d. Paralysis (hemiplegia/paraplegia/quadriplegia)

82. In which of the following layers of the skin is a network of nerve endings and blood vessels found?

a. Epidermis
b. Basement membrane (dermal-epidermal junction)
c. Dermis
d. Hypodermis (subcutaneous tissue)

83. Older patients are prone to dry skin primarily because:

a. They take less care of their skin.
b. Many medications are drying to the skin.
c. They have frequent skin infections.
d. Sweat glands begin to atrophy with age.

84. The thin skin typically seen in older adults is caused by:

a. Decreased thickness of the dermis
b. Decreased thickness of the epidermis
c. Decreased thickness of the hypodermis (subcutaneous tissue)
d. Mechanical irritation of the skin

85. Which of the following is the primary cause for skin failure?

a. Pressure
b. Xerosis
c. Incontinence
d. Hypoperfusion

86. If a patient failed to follow through with wound care and dressing changes as instructed by the healthcare provider, resulting in a deepening and infected wound, the type of negligence involved is:

a. Contributory negligence
b. Gross negligence
c. Negligent conduct
d. Comparative negligence

87. According to the Payne-Martin Classification System, a flap-type partial-thickness skin tear with 15% loss of epidermal flap is categorized as:

a. Category 1
b. Category 2
c. Category 3
d. Category 4

88. If a patient has developed 4 skin tears within the previous 90 days, according to the Skin Integrity Risk Assessment Tool, to which group does the patient belong?

a. Group I
b. Group II
c. Group III
d. Group IV

89. The Kennedy terminal ulcer phenomenon (rapid development of pressure injury in older adults nearing death) occurs most often in which of the following areas?

a. Elbow
b. Sacral
c. Calcaneous
d. Occipital

90. An immunocompromised patient develops a superficial infection on the left leg, spreading quickly with streaking, lymphedema, and clearly demarcated erythema and cellulitis. The patient experiences pain, moderate fever, and chills. These symptoms are consistent with:

a. Staphylococcal scaled skin syndrome
b. Candidiasis
c. Impetigo
d. Erysipelas

91. Which of the following is the appropriate initial response if a patient with paraplegia develops a pressure injury?

a. "What happened?"
b. "I'm so sorry this happened."
c. "Did you forget to shift your weight?"
d. "Let's figure out what you did wrong."

92. A solid skin barrier wafer with a pouch is applied to a copiously draining wound, but the skin beneath the wafer has become denuded. The best initial solution is to:

a. Apply a skin barrier powder to the denuded skin under the wafer.
b. Discontinue use of the pouch and apply topical dressing.
c. Apply a moisture barrier paste under the wafer.
d. Apply a moisture barrier ointment to the skin and absorbent dressings.

93. Which of the following biological skin substitutes would be appropriate for repair post-Mohs procedure for a large facial squamous cell carcinoma?

a. Apligraf
b. TransCyte
c. Integra
d. Dermagraft

94. During the phases of healing, which cell is responsible for beginning angiogenesis?

a. Neutrophil
b. Fibroblast
c. Macrophage
d. Myofibroblast

95. When educating a patient about preventing psoriasis flareups, the patient should be advised to:

a. Avoid hot, humid weather.
b. Use a dehumidifier.
c. Avoid sun exposure.
d. Apply moisturizers.

96. Which wound dressing type is most likely to result in pain during dressing change?

a. Gauze
b. Hydrocolloid
c. Hydrogel
d. Alginates

97. If an older patient has xerosis, tub baths should be limited to no more than:

a. 5 minutes
b. 10 minutes
c. 15 minutes
d. 20 minutes

98. How many days after injury does contraction of the wound usually begin?

a. 3
b. 5
c. 7
d. 9

99. Which of the following are risk factors for the development of biofilms?

a. Ischemia
b. Antibiotic therapy
c. Female gender
d. Age

100. Following removal of a hydrocolloid wafer, the healthcare provider notes a malodorous gel-like substance on the skin side of the dressing. This likely indicates:

a. A superficial infection
b. Improper positioning
c. A normal finding from exudate
d. Presence of a biofilm

101. A 54-year-old diabetic patient with heart disease developed a chronic (7 months duration) stage 4 coccygeal pressure injury following a stroke. The wound is large (7 × 5 × 1.5 cm) with copious exudate and signs of persistent infection. The best choice for wound care is to:

a. Pack with calcium alginate and cover with absorptive dressings.
b. Pack with cadexomer iodine beads and cover with bordered foam.
c. Apply a pouch to contain drainage.
d. Pack with silver alginate and cover with bordered foam.

102. A partial thickness wound typically heals within about:

a. 3–4 days
b. 7 days
c. 14 days
d. 30 days

103. If a patient has a full-thickness ulcer of the foot that extends down to the tendon but with no indications of abscess or osteomyelitis, this would be classified according to the Modified Wagner's Foot Ulcer Classification as:

a. Grade 2
b. Grade 3
c. Grade 4
d. Grade 5

104. To protect the feet of patients with peripheral neuropathy, what is the best emollient to apply to the feet?

a. Petrolatum jelly
b. Zinc oxide
c. Vicks VapoRub
d. Lotion

105. A patient has marked bilateral non-pitting edema of both lower legs and feet, including toes, and has thickening of the skin but no pigmentation. This edema can most likely be characterized as:

a. Orthostatic edema
b. Lymphedema
c. Lipedema
d. Chronic venous insufficiency

106. A patient has a wound infected with MRSA and is to receive treatment with ultraviolet light with a handheld device. At what distance from the wound should the ultraviolet light be held?

a. 1 inch
b. 4 inches
c. 8 inches
d. 12 inches

107. When using electrical stimulation (estim) for wound healing, treatments are usually carried out 5–6 days per week for:

a. 20–30 minutes
b. 30–45 minutes
c. 45–60 minutes
d. 60–90 minutes

108. A 5-year-old child has a series of bruises and lacerations in ovoid patterns suggesting bite injuries, which the parent states occurred when the child was playing with a toddler. Measurement of the intercanine distance is 3.2 cm, which indicates a likely bite from a(n):

a. Toddler
b. Older child
c. Adult
d. Person of any age

109. If a patient was bitten by a rattlesnake and develops pain and edema about the bite site and complains of perioral paresthesia, how many vials of antivenin are indicated?

a. 5 vials
b. 5–15 vials
c. 15–20 vials
d. 25 or more vials

110. After applying becaplermin (a growth factor) gel (Regranex) to a diabetic ulcer, the wound should be covered with:

a. Non-adherent dressing
b. Transparent film
c. Hydrogel wafer
d. Saline-moistened gauze

Answer Key and Explanation

1. D: The three wound factors that most often lead to social isolation are:

- **Malodor**: Patients may feel embarrassed or ashamed if the wound has a foul odor and may avoid contact with others when they encounter negative attitudes. In turn, others may avoid contact with the patients, increasing their isolation.
- **Drainage**: Trying to cope with drainage in social situations can be difficult, especially if patients are worried that the dressing may become saturated and leak and that drainage may soak into clothing and furnishings.
- **Visible wound:** Wounds that are disfiguring or easily seen, especially wounds on the face or other visible parts of the body, often result in negative responses from others.

2. C: If a patient with peripheral arterial disease develops an ulcer on the foot, vascular laboratory/imaging studies (such as arteriograms and Doppler ultrasounds) are indicated to help determine if the ulcer resulted from ischemia or pressure, since both may be implicated to some degree. The degree of circulatory impairment must be assessed in order to determine the best approach to treatment and to prevent further breakdown of tissue. If circulatory impairment is severe, prevention of pressure ulcers is challenging.

3. D: If a 65-year-old patient's zinc level is 60 mcg/dL, the anticipated effect on the patient's wound is delayed healing. Zinc is essential to the enzymes involved in metabolism of proteins and carbohydrates and is also involved in DNA replication. About 20% of the body's zinc is stored within the skin. Normal values for adults are 70–120 mcg/dL. Zinc levels must be monitored, especially with large wounds such as burn injuries, and supplementation provided if levels fall below normal.

4. A: Ultrasound is used in wound care to stimulate healing and debride wounds. It produces mechanical vibration and may be used with or without heat. Ultrasound is most effective on collagen-based tissues, such as tendons, ligaments, and fascia. High frequency ultrasound (0.5–3 MHz) is used primarily to stimulate healing and to deliver transdermal medications. Penetration depth correlates with frequency: 1.0 MHz ultrasound can penetrate up to 5 cm, making it suitable for deeper injuries, while 3 MHz ultrasound penetrates 1–2 cm and is typically used to treat superficial skin lesions. Low frequency ultrasound (20–50 kHz) may be used to debride necrotic tissue and promote healing and may have an antibacterial effect.

5. C: Occlusive dressings should keep the wound warm and moist. Reasons include:

- Reduction in dehydration allows cells such as neutrophils and fibroblasts to carry out their functions in wound repair. This also results in less cell death.
- Angiogenesis requires a moist environment and low oxygen tension.
- Autolytic debridement with proteolytic enzymes is enhanced.
- Re-epithelization of tissue occurs because the epidermal cells are able to spread across the surface of the wound.
- Reduction in microorganisms, facilitated by the seal provided by occlusive dressings, decreases infection.
- Pain reduction results from the protection of nerve endings and the need for fewer dressing changes.

6. B: The best candidate for hyperbaric oxygen therapy is the patient with chronic diabetic ulcers (Wagner classification III or higher), refractory to standard treatment. During treatment, patients breathe 100% oxygen in a pressurized environment. Hyperbaric oxygen therapy increases available oxygen to tissues by 10–20 times. Blood that is saturated increases perfusion of the tissues. Hyperbaric oxygen therapy is indicated for peripheral arterial insufficiency, compromised skin from grafts, and diabetic ulcers (usually Wagner III or higher). In 2003, Medicare approved payment for hyperbaric oxygen therapy to treat diabetic ulcers.

7. A: Sharp debridement with saucerization (tissue excavated to form a shallow depression to facilitate drainage) is the best choice for an infected diabetic ulcer with callus formation, although repeat saucerization may be required with each dressing change. All of the callus and necrotic tissue should be removed and the wound flushed with sterile saline. In some cases, autolytic debridement with hydrocolloids or hydrogels may be used first to help soften the callus prior to its removal.

8. B: The pinch test is not very reliable for assessing dehydration, especially if done over areas with much subcutaneous tissue, so the best sites are on the forehead or over the sternum. Indications of dehydration include cracked lips, dry mucous membranes, tachycardia, altered sensations, hypotension, and weight loss. If dehydration is suspected, then it should be confirmed with diagnostic testing, such as serum osmolality, serum sodium, BUN, BUN/creatinine ration, urine specific gravity, and albumin.

9. B: A full-thickness ulcer that extends to the tendon or joint but without abscess or osteomyelitis is classified as Grade 2. The Modified Wagner Foot Ulcer Classification System separates foot ulcers into 6 grades (Grade 0 to Grade 5). Classification is based on depth of lesion, presence of osteomyelitis, gangrene, infection, ischemia, and neuropathy but does not include ulcer size, so this grading system is not used in isolation; however, it is predictive of outcomes, with grades 3–4 indicating marked compromise.

10. C: Transparent film should be changed every 3–5 days, although the dressing should always be changed if leakage occurs, as this can cause tissue maceration. Transparent film is most useful for dry eschar, which should be crosshatched prior to application of the film to facilitate autolysis. The dressing should be at least 2 inches larger than the size of the wound. The wound should be irrigated with NS and a skin sealant applied to surrounding tissue prior to application of the dressing.

11. B: Chronic ulcers with poor perfusion or other complicating factors, such as infection, may remain in the inflammatory phase of healing. If the macrophages that are activated during the inflammation stage are not able to adequately attract fibroblasts, then the angiogenesis, formation of collagen, and epithelization that are necessary for the wound to heal do not take place, so the wound remains stalled for long periods of time unless the complicating factors are aggressively treated and reversed.

12. A: Hypertrophic scars most frequently occur over joints where there is tension on the wound. They remain localized to the area of the original wound and may spontaneously regress. They may result in contracture of the wound. **Keloid scars** most frequently occur on the upper back and chest as well as the deltoids and earlobes. They extend beyond the original wound and rarely regress. They usually arise after the wound has healed as raised, shiny, rope-like fibrous scars. They do not result in contracture of the wound.

13. D: Behavioral outcomes should always be measurable, such as "Able to demonstrate dressing change in 3 days." This outcome covers a specific task and a time frame, making it easy to evaluate. Words such as *understands*, *accepts*, and *feels* are not measurable. Behavioral outcomes should be described in terms of actions words, such as *demonstrates*, *states*, *describes*, and *lists*. Behavioral outcomes should always be things that can be directly observed and measured to determine if outcomes have been successfully achieved within the allotted time.

14. C: If a 15-year-old patient was attacked by a dog and has severe contaminated bite wounds on the legs, the wound will likely be debrided, and closure will likely take place through tertiary healing (healing by third intention), leaving the wound open because of the risk of infection. When the wound begins to heal and the risk of infection decreases, the wound may be surgically closed or covered with a skin graft. Puncture wounds and animal bites carry a high risk for infection and are often left open to prevent formation of abscesses.

15. A: The most common cause of venous outflow obstruction and venous ulceration is deep vein thrombosis. With obstruction, veins distal to the obstructed area become distended, resulting in increased venous hypertension (sustained increased pressure in the legs). As the venous pressure rises, venous stasis occurs, leading to ulceration. Other factors that can also contribute to increased venous hypertension include obesity, CHF, edema, trauma, ascites, and tumors of the legs.

16. B: An Unna boot is used to treat non-healing stasis ulcers in ambulatory patients. If the ulcer is draining, it should be packed with alginate, and a dressing should be applied to absorb the discharge until the Unna boot is changed. Before applying, the leg and ulcers should be cleaned, and the leg should be patted dry. Most wraps contain a moisture barrier, generally, zinc oxide and glycerin. The wrap must be applied upward from the toes to about 1 inch below the knee. It is then covered with an elastic bandage or self-adhering bandage (such as Coban), stretched to 50% tension.

17. D: The best choice for a patient with large stage III and stage IV pressure injuries on multiple turning sites is a low air loss therapy device. Low air loss devices may use a bed frame or be placed on top of a standard mattress. Low air loss therapy devices have low moisture retention, reduced heat accumulation, and provide relief of pressure in any position, so they are particularly useful for patients with multiple pressure injuries. The devices comprise connected air-filled pillows covered by a low-friction material. The amount of air and pressure in each pillow can be separately calibrated.

18. C: Foreign material should be removed by hand debridement from a large open contaminated wound, followed by large-volume irrigation at 5–8 lb. pressure per square inch (usually using a <19-gauge needle) and pulsatile lavage, in order to reduce the risk of infection. Pulsatile high-pressure lavage is irrigation of an infected or necrotic wound under pressure, using an electrically powered device. Normal saline is commonly used for lavage treatments, with the amount varying according to the size and amount of exudate on the wound. It is recommended that pressure be between 8–15 psi.

19. A: Bioburden refers to the presence of necrotic tissue and debris that prevent epithelialization from occurring. Bioburden contributes to the development of infection in the wound. **Contamination** of a wound means that bacteria are present but are not multiplying. **Colonization** is common and occurs when bacteria multiply in the wound but do not cause an inflammatory response, damage tissues, or retard healing. **Critical colonization** occurs when bacteria replicate to a level that causes delay in healing without causing an inflammatory response or an infection with tissue damage.

20. C: Undermining, which is damaged tissue under intact skin, usually occurs around the perimeter of a wound. Undermining is reported in centimeters and in relation to the open wound by reference to a clock face: "Extends 1.8 cm width from 1 o'clock to 4 o'clock." If the undermining is open, it can be measured by insertion of a sterile swab. In some cases, tissue may be damaged but remains intact; in that case, undermining is estimated by palpation as undermined tissue may feel spongy.

21. B: The increased airflow with fluidized air/high-air-loss support surfaces can increase evaporative fluid loss, so patients must be adequately hydrated to compensate and avoid dehydration. Intake and output must be carefully monitored, and skin turgor and mucous membranes must be evaluated. Fluidized air/high-air-loss support surfaces have beads with a pH of 10 (alkaline), so they have bacteriocidal properties, decreasing risk of infection. These support surfaces reduce friction, shear, and pressure as well as moisture, decreasing risk of fungal infection.

22. C: Because enzymes require a moist environment, the first step when treating dry eschar is to crosshatch through the outer layers of the eschar. Chemical debridement with enzymes, such as collagenase and papain/urea, is effective for wounds with necrosis and eschar but may take several days to several weeks to debride a large area of eschar. Various types of dressing can be used with enzymes, but they must be easily removable because enzymes must be applied one to two times daily.

23. D: ABI scoring interpretation is detailed below. The score of 0.75 is associated with severe disease, ischemia.

ABI scoring	
>1.3	Abnormally high, may indicate calcification of vessel wall
1–1.1	Normal reading, asymptomatic
<0.95	Indicates narrowing of one or more leg blood vessels
<0.8	Moderate, often associated with intermittent claudication during exercise
≤0.6–0.8	Borderline perfusion
0.5–0.75	Severe disease, ischemia
<0.5	Pain, even at rest, limb threatened
0.25	Critical limb-threatening condition

24. B: Painless open ulcers on the pressure areas on the bottom of the foot surrounded by calloused skin indicate neuropathic ulcers, such as those commonly found with diabetic polyneuropathy. Because of reduced sensation, patients may develop ulcers from chronic pressure (indicated by the callus formation) without noticing, especially if they do not check their feet or are unable to do so. The nylon monofilament test can be used to assess the patient's degree of protective sensation.

25. B: Instrumental Activities of Daily Living (IADL): An assessment tool to measure 8 activities necessary for an adult to function independently. This tool helps to determine the need for supportive services. **Barthel Index of Activities of Daily Living**: Assesses the functional ability of older adults in 10 categories. It is used to assess the person's disabilities and need for assistance. **Index of Independence of Activities of Daily Living (Katz Index):** Evaluates 6 areas to provide an assessment of the person's need for assistance and progression of disease and/or disability. **Palliative Performance Scale:** Assesses the functional ability of older adults receiving palliative care.

26. C: If a patient in a hospital that is part of the in-patient prospective payment system has a stage 3 pressure injury present on admission, but this was neither identified nor documented, the hospital cannot claim payment for the pressure injury as a primary or secondary diagnosis. For this reason, a careful physical examination and documentation of findings must be completed on admission because failing to do so may result in reduced payment, as the pressure injury may be classified as a hospital-acquired condition.

27. A: Support surface material should provide at least an inch of support under areas to be protected when in use to prevent "bottoming out." When determining the type of overlay, the patient's size and weight must be considered. Generally, all patients at risk should have some type of pressure-reducing overlay on their beds. Visco-elastic foam provides some protection and may protect from shear and friction. Other non-dynamic overlays, such as those made with foam chips, tend to deteriorate faster than visco-elastic foam.

28. B: Increased protein is especially important for wound healing. The average healthy person requires about 0.8 g of protein per kilogram every day (40–70 g). However, if a person has a wound, not only must the person have adequate calories and general nutrition, but also daily added protein and vitamins as well. Protein amounts are increased to 1.25–2.0 g per kilogram to promote healing. Healing requires extra calories as well, but ensuring a high protein nutritious diet is more important than simply reducing calories or fat or increasing carbohydrates.

29. B: An example of a condition/situation that is covered by the CMS surgical dressing benefit is a stage 2 pressure injury. Non-covered conditions/situations include first-degree burns, stage 1 pressure injuries, venipuncture/arterial puncture sites (for blood sampling), skin tears, abrasions, and draining cutaneous fistula not caused/treated by surgery. Criteria for inclusion include dressings that are medically necessary because a wound was caused by surgery or treated with surgery or dressings that are medically necessary because the wound requires debridement.

30. D: Wounds that involve full-thickness skin loss with margins that cannot be approximated and/or have non-viable wound edges are usually left to heal by secondary intention. In some cases of large wounds, skin grafting may be required. Secondary intention healing is also indicated for grossly contaminated wounds that carry a high risk of infection and necrotic tissue. The wound is covered with a dressing and left to heal through regeneration rather than repair, resulting in scar tissue and contraction.

31. A: Prealbumin is used to assess acute changes in nutritional status, so a decrease from 16 mg/dL to 10 mg/dL indicates that the patient has recent acute inadequate protein intake, possibly because of the increased demand for protein and calories to promote healing. Because prealbumin's half-life is only 2–3 days, it can change rapidly in response to nutritional changes:

- Normal value: 16–40 mg/dL
- Mild deficiency: 10–15mg/dL
- Moderate deficiency: 5–9 mg/dL
- Severe deficiency: <5 mg/dL

This patient's diet should be re-evaluated, and protein and calories increased to meet the increased needs.

32. B: Patients taking oral iron should also take vitamin C because it increases the iron absorption. Dosage is usually equivalent to or higher than the iron dosage. Vitamin C also promotes the formation of collagen and promotes wound healing, so deficiency can result in impaired healing and increased capillary fragility. Ferrous sulfate is usually used for iron deficiency in adults, with dosage varying according to hemoglobin and other factors. Patients should receive nutritional counseling regarding foods high in iron and vitamin C.

33. D: Because injury to tissues may be more extensive than what is visible with a pressure injury, a pressure injury in which the base cannot be visualized must be staged as "Unstageable" with the NPIAP Pressure Injury Staging until the wound can be adequately debrided and the base examined to determine depth. The base may be obscured by slough of various colors (yellow to brown) or eschar (brown or black). To ensure proper treatment, a wound classified as unstageable should be debrided and restaged as soon as possible.

34. C: Wounds should be irrigated with pressures of 10–15 psi. An irrigation pressure of <4 psi does not adequately cleanse a wound, and pressures >15 psi can result in trauma to the wound, interfering with healing. A mechanical irrigation device is more effective for irrigation than a bulb syringe, which delivers about ≤2 psi. A 250 mL squeeze bottle supplies about 4.5 psi, which is adequate for low-pressure cleaning. A 35-mL syringe with a 19-gauge needle provides about 8 psi.

35. D: Transmission-based precautions include:

Contact	Use personal protective equipment (PPE), including gown and gloves, for all contacts with the patient or patient's immediate environment. Maintain patient in private room or >3 feet away from other patients.
Droplet	Use mask while caring for the patient. Maintain patient in a private room or > 3 feet away from other patients with curtain separating them. Use patient mask if transporting patient from one area to another.
Airborne	Place patient in an airborne infection isolation room. Use ≥N95 respirators (or masks) while caring for patient.

36. A: Charcot's arthropathy should be treated with total contact cast for months, with duration depending on the location of the deformity: 12 months for hindfoot, 9 months for midfoot, and 6 months for forefoot. The casts should be changed weekly during the time the volume is changing and then every 2–3 weeks. Temperatures should be checked on both sides and should be within 3 degrees Fahrenheit after recalcification. The patient may be allowed gradual weight bearing after skin has resumed normal temperature.

37. C: The only way to prevent pressure on the heels is to elevate the heel so that it is not in contact with a surface, such as the bed or wheelchair footrest. A special heel elevation device can be utilized, or a pillow may be placed under the legs to elevate the heels. Additionally, a pillow should be placed between the ankles to prevent pressure injuries where the feet contact each other. The patient's position should be changed frequently with full-body turning to 30-degree lateral position, avoiding side-lying.

38. C: Because shear results from a combination of friction and pressure, the only safe way to avoid shear when moving a patient up in bed is to use a lift/turning sheet with two people lifting and moving the patient toward the head of the bed. If possible, the patient can assist by utilizing a trapeze, but the patient should avoid pulling himself/herself toward the head of the bed with the trapeze unless the patient is able to lift completely off the bed with the feet placed flat on the bed to avoid shear on the heels.

39. A: Venous dermatitis appears on the ankles and lower legs and can cause severe itching and pain, and without treatment to control the dermatitis, it may deteriorate, causing ulcers to form, so treatment is needed to alleviate the symptoms. Initial treatment is usually with topical antihistamines. If this does not relieve symptoms, then low dose topical steroids may be used for short periods only (2 weeks) to reduce inflammation and itching because of the danger of increasing ulceration.

40. D: Metronidazole, in gel or solution, has proven to be an effective topical treatment to control infection and odor in necrotic tumors as it is effective against a wide range of anaerobic bacteria. The solution is used to irrigate the wound, and the gel is applied directly to the tissue. Hydrogen peroxide may irritate the tissue, while Dakin's solution has an odor that some patient's dislike, although both may reduce tumor odor. Some people have used yogurt and buttermilk topically to reduce odor by reducing wound pH, but there is little research to support their use.

41. B: Troughing is one method of fistula management that is appropriate for fistulas in the posterior aspect of an abdominal wound; however, this technique does not protect the wound from exudate, so the wound can become contaminated. Troughing involves applying skin barrier wafer to the skin surrounding the wound and skin barrier paste to the edges. Then, thin film dressing is applied to the wound down to the fistula opening, and an ostomy pouch is cut to fit and applied about the fistula opening. This method allows drainage from the wound and the fistula to mix as they both drain into the ostomy appliance.

42. C: The healing ridge, which is the result of collagen deposition that begins in the inflammatory stage and continues to the proliferation stage, should be evident directly under a suture line between days 5 and 9 after suturing. If the healing ridge is missing, then the wound is at increased risk of dehiscence and infection. The healing ridge appears as an area of induration extending about 1 cm on both sides of the wound.

43. D: Elbow and heel pads do not prevent pressure injuries but they do reduce friction, which can lead to skin breakdown. Friction occurs when body parts rub against the sheet or each other. Elbow pads are especially useful for patients who exhibit repetitive movements of the arms. Other methods to reduce friction include applying transparent film, skin sealant, or other protective dressings such as a thin hydrocolloid or other padding to vulnerable skin sites.

44. C: When cleansing a wound in a shower, the showerhead should be about 12 inches away from the wound. The showerhead may be covered with a clean washcloth or other cloth if necessary, to reduce the water pressure. Showering should usually be done over 5–10 minutes to ensure that the wound is adequately clean. The patient may be seated in a shower chair if standing is difficult or the wound is in a hard to reach area.

45. A: High-level compression therapy should exert 30–40 mmHg at the ankle. Low level products exert ≤23 mmHg at the ankle. Static compression utilizes various products (layered wraps, single-layer wraps, and compression stockings) to apply gradually increasing pressure to the lower extremity, distally-to-proximally (usually beginning at the foot or ankle and extending to the knee). The primary purpose is to prevent venous ulceration or further deterioration of existing ulcers.

46. D: Ayello's ASSESSMENTS:

A	Anatomic location and age of wound
S	Size, shape, and stage (NPIAP for pressure injury or Wagner for neurotropic)
S	Sinus tract, tunneling, undermining, and fistulae
E	Exudate (amount, consistency, and color)
S	Sepsis
S	Surrounding skin
M	Maceration
E	Edges and epithelialization
N	Necrotic tissue

T	Tissue bed and tenderness (0–10 scale for pain)
S	Status of wound and supportive therapy

47. B: Because exposure to air will kill anaerobic bacteria, a culture should be taken with a syringe without the needle. The healthcare provider should insert the tip of the syringe as deeply into the wound as possible, aspirating 2–3 mL of exudate. Immediately after removing the syringe from the wound, the nurse should attach a needle, expel all air from the syringe, and inject the exudate into a special sealed culture tube intended for anaerobic organisms. Aerobic organisms are cultured by swabbing the wound surface with a sterile swab.

48. D: Malnutrition risk factors:

- Hypermetabolism resulting from various diseases
- Weight loss, especially sudden or loss of 10% of normal weight over a 3-month period
- Low body weight of <90% of ideal body weight for age or low Body Mass Index (BMI) <18.5
- Immunosuppressive drugs that interfere with nutrient absorption, malabsorption of nutrients caused by diseases, changes in appetite, and food intolerances, such as lactose intolerance
- Dietary restrictions, such as limiting of protein with kidney failure
- Functional limitations, such as inability to feed oneself
- Lack of teeth or dentures, limiting intake
- Alterations of taste or smell that render food unpalatable

49. A: Extrinsic factors are those that derive from outside the body, such as wound bioburden. Other extrinsic factors include radiotherapy, medications, interfering therapies, and stress. Intrinsic factors are those that are inherent in the patient and can include the patient's age, disease (such as diabetes), immunosuppression (from disease, such as HIV/AIDS, or from medications, such as chemotherapeutic agents). Malnutrition and neuropathy are also intrinsic factors that can affect healing.

50. C: NPWT is intended for wounds healing by second or third intention, so the best candidate would be a stage III pressure injury. NPWT reduces edema, promotes healing, and decreases exudate but is contraindicated with exposed blood vessels, osteomyelitis, and exposed organs. For NPWT, the wound bed is filled with nonadherent porous foam and secured by occlusive transparent film into which an opening is cut over the foam and a drainage tube applied. This tube is then attached to a suction canister to create a closed system.

51. D: The clock method, which involves measuring the wound from 12 o'clock to 6 o'clock and from 9 o'clock to 3 o'clock, always tracks the same site, while the GLBGW method may involve measurements at different sites each time because wounds often don't heal evenly. The clock method does require more precision to ensure that measurements are exactly perpendicular to each other. The GLBGW method is the most commonly used, but studies show it often overestimates the wound surface, while the clock method may be more accurate, but both methods can overestimate to some degree because of wound irregularities.

52. D: When testing the VPT, the nurse should first conduct a preliminary test on the patient's sternum so that the patient knows what sensation to expect. During the test, the patient should keep the eyes closed and should report when first feeling a vibratory sensation and when it ceases. After striking the tuning fork, it is applied to the dorsum of the great toe (proximal to the nail bed) with the test repeated 8 times. A patient receives one point each time he/she fails to feel the vibration, so scores range from 0 (good) to 8 (impaired).

53. C: Immobility is the primary risk factor for development of pressure injuries, although inactivity and sensory loss are also contributing factors. People with sensory loss may not feel the discomfort that occurs with pressure. Studies have indicated that those who make 50 spontaneous movements during the night have almost no risk of developing a pressure injury, while those who make 20 or fewer spontaneous movements during the night are at high risk, highlighting the importance of frequent repositioning of patients whose mobility is limited.

54. D: Muscle tissue and granulation tissue may be similar in color, and location alone is not adequate to differentiate the two. Because muscle tissue is firmer and reacts differently to pressure, the best method to differentiate the two is to palpate and gently pinch the tissue. Granulation tissue tends to be soft and spongy and will often bleed if disturbed, such as by gently pinching. Muscle tissue, however, is more resilient to pressure but may twitch if pinched or palpated.

55. A: Pulsed lavage with suction (PLWS) is the best choice as it is effective in reducing bacterial load and can be used with undermining and tunneling. Additionally, it can be carried out effectively at bedside if necessary. Whirlpool is contraindicated in febrile patients and cannot be carried out if the patient is undergoing cardiac monitoring. Wet-to-dry dressings are no longer recommended as they may damage new tissue. Flushing a large contaminated wound with a 35 mL syringe and 19-gauge needle is likely to be ineffective.

56. B: The five Ps of neurovascular assessment are:

- Pain: amount and severity and contributing factors
- Pallor: indicates decreased arterial supply
- Pulselessness: note weak or absent pulses; capillary refill time should be ≤3 seconds
- Paresthesia: numbness, tingling
- Paraplegia: assess motion

57. B: The normal phasic flow pattern is triphasic when assessing peripheral pulses with continuous wave Doppler (representing systolic forward flow, negative deflection during diastole, and return to forward flow). As the artery loses the ability to recoil, such as through atherosclerosis, the phasic flow pattern changes to biphasic and then eventually to monophasic when the pulsatile nature of the blood flow is impaired. Continuous wave Doppler is most often used when calculating the ankle-brachial index (ABI).

58. A: The best debridement choice for a venous ulcer with hard brown adherent eschar covering 60% of the wound is autolytic with hydrogels. Because of the edema associated with venous ulcers, they tend to produce a lot of exudate, and this increases as the wound debrides. Therefore, hydrogel dressings, which have absorptive properties, help to contain the exudate and prevent maceration of the surrounding tissue. Enzymatic debridement may also be used, but the surrounding skin must be monitored carefully and protected from the enzyme and exudate.

59. D: Upon application of Apligraf to the wound, it appears similar to a skin graft, but after about a week, it should appear gelatinous, so this is a normal transition, and care must be taken not to disrupt or wash away the biological skin substitute for the first 2–3 weeks. In some cases, reapplication is necessary. Apligraf is supplied in a thermally-controlled container and requires incubation prior to application. Apligraf is applied to the wound surface (edges overlapping) and covered with a compression wrap to secure.

60. C: Soaking dressing to loosen prior to removal relieves cyclic acute pain. CWPE model:

- Non-cyclic acute wound pain: Occurs with trauma, such as sharp debridement. Interventions include topical or local anesthetics and anti-anxiety medication.
- Cyclic acute wound pain: Occurs at regular times, such as with wound changes or position changes. Interventions include soaking dressing, timeouts, non-adherent dressings, and use of repositioning devices.
- Chronic wound pain: Occurs continuously. Interventions include heat, transcutaneous nerve stimulation, and tricyclic antidepressants.

61. B: Indications of limb ischemia include ankle pressure <40 mmHg and toe pressure <30 mmHg. Critical limb ischemia occurs when resting pain is so severe it requires analgesia for more than 2 weeks duration. Limb ischemia can result in impaired healing of arterial ulcers and increased wound pain. Pain may be evident on positional changes (increasing with elevation, decreasing with dependency), when walking (usually relieved after about 10 minutes rest), or at rest with limb elevated (neuropathic).

62. B: High compression stockings, class IV (50–60 mmHg), are recommended only for edema associated with lymphedema, which is characterized by edema that begins soft and pitting but over time becomes firm and diffuse but more severe distally than proximally. It often occurs bilaterally and is usually not associated with pain, although the patient may complain the affected limbs feel heavy. Ulcerations are rare, and elevation provides only partial relief. Skin eventually thickens and tissue becomes fibrotic.

63. A: Warm mineral oil treatment for one week during the night can relieve dry, scaly, pruritic skin associated with peripheral edema. The legs are washed and dried thoroughly, and then warm mineral oil is applied to all affected areas (usually from the toes to the knees). The skin is then covered with plastic wrap and secured over the feet with cotton stockings. The plastic wrap is removed in the morning, and the skin is washed and dried, followed by application of a thick moisturizing cream.

64. D: While all of these are attributes of foam dressings, amorphous hydrogels and alginates are used to contain wounds with a large amount of exudate. Foam dressings are highly absorbant and thermally insulating, so the primary purpose of covering these wound fillers with foam dressing is to absorb additional exudate and to raise the core temperature of the wound in order to promote autolysis. Additionally, foam dressings conform to the body and can easily mold to irregular body surfaces.

65. C: Hypertonic sodium chloride may be applied to a wound to reduce hypergranulation as it is less toxic than silver nitrate. Hypergranulation, which inhibits epithelialization, often occurs in wounds left open to heal by secondary intention. Hypertonic sodium chloride dressings are applied daily until the granulation level is normal but should be changed every 24 hours to inspect the wound. The hypertonic saline in the dressing draws excess fluid from the cells on the wound surface.

66. B: Hydrocolloids or film dressings are the best choices to provide protection to reddened skin and prevent further skin deterioration as they reduce friction and shear. **Foam dressings** are used for moist wounds with exudate. **Sheet hydrogel** is used to rehydrate slough to aide in autolysis, so it is useful when slough is present with minimal exudate. **Silver dressings** have antibacterial properties and are used to treat infected wounds or, as in the case of burns, to prevent infection.

67. A: Procedure for lidocaine soak:

1. Draw 5–10 mL of 2% lidocaine into a syringe.
2. Remove wound dressing and cleanse wound.
3. Place clean dry gauze over surface of wound.
4. Saturate the wound area (and gauze) with the 2% lidocaine.
5. Allow the lidocaine solution to contact the wound for 3–5 minutes.
6. Evaluate pain sensation to ensure the area is anesthetized.
7. Debride wound and redress as appropriate.

68. B: Wounds that take fewer than 14 days to heal are often partial thickness wounds that heal with no or minimal scarring, but the potential for scarring is greater for those that take more than 14 days. Pressure dressings or garments are used commonly with burns, and special pressure garments in various sizes are available for different parts of the body. In small areas, such as on a forearm, pressure dressings may be applied with self-adherent stretch wrap or tubular dressings.

69. C: When exercising and stretching a scar, maximal stretch is usually indicated by blanching of the scar. While some pain is often involved in stretching, it should not exceed the patient's tolerance. Slow stretching that is sustained is better than rapid stretching and relaxing exercises. Exercises to stretch scars should be individually determined and depend on the type of scar, location of scar, and phase of healing as well as patient factors, such as age, mobility, cognition, and medical status.

70. D: Signs of inflammation are usually evident in the acute surgical wound for the first 4 days, and this is a normal finding. Indications can include increased skin temperature about the incision, erythema, and edema. If no evidence of inflammation occurs, then this may indicate immunosuppression. Because hair follicles are usually present, epithelium resurfaces the incision within 72 hours, providing protection from bacteria and mild trauma, although the tensile strength of the healing incision remains weak.

71. C: Moderate risk (65–90%) The Braden scale rates 5 areas (Sensory perception, moisture, activity, mobility, and usual nutrition pattern) with a 1–4 scale and one area (friction and shear) with a 1–3 scale. Lower scores indicate increased risk. The scores for all six items are totaled, and a risk assigned according to the number:

- 23 (best score): excellent prognosis, very minimal risk
- 15–18: mild risk (50–60%) with 16 usually being the breakpoint for pressure injury
- 13–14: moderate risk (65–90%)
- 10–12: high risk (90–100%) with 6 the worst score

72. D: Pillows are useful for reducing tissue compression, especially to protect the heels, even when using support surfaces. Pillow bridging usually requires placement of at least 5 pillows with one in each of the following positions: under the legs (to protect the heels), between the ankles, between the knees, behind the back, and underneath the head. An additional small pillow may be used to support the upper arm when the patient is lying in a side-lying tilt.

73. C: The venous refill time procedure begins with asking the patient to lie supine for a few moments and then having the patient elevate the legs to 45 degrees for one minute. Next, the patient is assisted into sitting position with the feet dependent while the nurse closely observes the veins on the dorsum of the foot and counts the seconds before normal filling. Normal venous refill time is 5–15 seconds, and venous occlusion is indicated with times >20 seconds.

74. A: Because these findings (swelling, drainage, pain, and purple color) are consistent with wet gangrene, no debridement should be carried out. The patient should be referred to a surgeon immediately. Wet gangrene involves necrosis of tissue from excessive moisture and bacterial infection, causing bacterial gases to accumulate in the damaged tissue. Dry gangrene occurs from impaired circulation, resulting in dry, black, shriveled tissue.

75. C: The Harris mat, used for pressure testing, is a tool that indicates the patient's plantar pressure and weight distribution and can be used to provide a pattern for off-loading. The mat is placed on the floor and opened, and ink is applied with a roller to the impression side. Then, a piece of paper is placed on the other half of the mat. The impression side is folded over to cover the paper (ink side down). Then, the patient steps onto the impression side, and the ink transfers onto the paper, with darker areas indicating areas of higher pressure.

76. D: Patients with peripheral neuropathy should have professional skin and nail care of the foot at least monthly so that the foot can be thoroughly examined and assessed in order to prevent ulceration. Those with poor hygiene or compromised tissue may need care more frequently. Toenails grow at the rate of about 1 mm per month while fingernails grow at the rate of about 3 mm per month. Toenails should be cut straight across with sharp corners smoothed with a file. Patients should be taught proper hygiene and care of the feet.

77. B: If 6 months after an artificial hip was implanted the patient develops an infection of the fascia and muscle layers and purulent discharge, the wound would be categorized according to the CDC's Categories of Surgical Wound Infections as Category 2, deep incisional. Category 2 surgical wound infections are those that occur within 30 days (if no implant) or within a year (with implant) and involve the fascia and muscle layers with one further indication, including purulent discharge, positive wound culture, wound dehiscence, abscess, and/or physician diagnosis.

78. B: For the purpose of Medicare reimbursement for home healthcare, working 2 days a week in an office would disqualify a patient from being considered homebound. Criteria include the need for supportive devices (such as walker or wheelchair), the need for special transportation services, the need for assistance from others, a condition that requires the patient to stay within the home (such as a contagious disorder), and a condition in which the symptoms (such as pain) worsen if the patient leaves the home.

79. D: The data set that is part of essential wound documentation in skilled nursing facilities is the Minimum Data Set. The MDS requires that patients admitted to CMS certified skilled nursing facilities undergo a comprehensive assessment of health condition and functional capabilities. The assessment must be done on admission, when changes in conditions occur, and on a regularly scheduled basis every 3 months. The assessment includes cognitive status, functional ability, behavioral status, and psychosocial functioning as well as evidence of geriatric syndromes (pain, incontinence, impaired nutrition) and wishes for life care.

80. A: TcPO2 level <20 mmHg usually indicates that a wound will not heal because oxygen supply is inadequate, while a level >30 mmHg indicates good potential for healing, and the wound can be safely debrided. The transcutaneous method is contraindicated if edema or infection is present in the wound as results will not be accurate. Depending on the type of machine for testing, the TcPO2 can take up to 30 minutes to complete.

81. B: According to the NPIAP consensus statement, the patient circumstance that may result in unavoidable pressure injuries is hemodynamic instability that prevents repositioning. Other conditions include skin failure and patient refusal to turn or reposition. Patients at risk should be placed on pressure-distributing surfaces (mattresses, chair cushions) before skin begins to break down. While standard practice is to reposition patients every 2 hours, some patients may require more frequent repositioning and assessment of skin.

82. C: A network of nerve endings and blood vessels is found in the dermis layer (which lies between the basement membrane and the hypodermis) of the skin. The dermis is itself composed of two layers: papillary dermis and reticular dermis. Sweat glands, sebaceous glands, and hair follicles are also found in the dermis, which provides structure and strength to the skin, provides moisture, and helps to resist shearing. The dermis is essential in providing nourishment (blood, oxygen, nutrients) to the skin.

83. D: Older patients are prone to dry skin primarily because sweat glands begin to atrophy with age as part of the normal aging process. As the glands shrink in size, they produce less perspiration and are less sensitive to temperature changes. Perspiration is important to thermoregulation and skin hydration. As perspiration decreases, the skin tends to become looser (taking on a sagging appearance) and dry, making it more vulnerable to infection and mechanical trauma.

84. A: The thin skin typically seen in older adults is caused by decreased thickness of the dermis, which results in fewer collagen fibers, blood vessels, and nerve endings. This, in turn, results in decreased sensation and thermoregulation and impaired fluid retention, giving the skin a sagging appearance. The thinner skin is more at risk for injuries from shear and pressure, and wounds tend to heal more slowly. Over time, the basement membrane flattens, and the epidermis thins as well.

85. D: The primary cause for skin failure is hypoperfusion, usually associated with severe systemic dysfunction or multi-organ failure at the end of life. With skin failure, skin breakdown and pressure injuries may occur without pressure because the impaired circulation makes the skin more susceptible to injury. However, it can be difficult to differentiate a lesion associated with skin failure from a pressure injury. Skin failure may be acute (associated with critical illness), chronic (associated with chronic illness), or end-stage (associated with end-of-life).

86. A: Types of negligence include:

- Negligent conduct: An individual failed to provide reasonable care or to protect/assist another, based on standards and expertise.
- Gross negligence: An individual willfully provided inadequate care while disregarding the safety and security of another.
- Contributory negligence: The injured party contributed to their own harm.
- Comparative negligence: Individuals involved are assessed for the percentage of negligence attributed to each.

87. B: According to the Payne-Martin Classification System (3 categories only), a flap-type partial-thickness skin tear with 15% loss of epidermal flap is categorized as category 2—scant tissue loss.

- Category 1 includes skin tear (linear full-thickness or flap partial-thickness) leaving avulsed skin adequate to cover wound. Tears may be linear or flap-type.
- Category 2 (as above) also includes moderate to large tissue loss type with more than 25% loss of epidermal flap.
- Category 3 includes skin tear with complete loss of tissue, involving a partial-thickness wound with no epidermal flap.

88. A: If a patient has developed 4 skin tears (or ANY skin tears) within the previous 90 days, according to the Skin Integrity Risk Assessment Tool, the patient belongs to Group I and should have implementation of a skin tear risk prevention plan. Groups II and III include multiple risk factors that may increase incidence of skin tears although the patient's skin remains intact. Group II includes impaired decision-making, impaired vision, requiring assistance with ADLs/wheelchair, poor balance, being confined to chair bed, impaired gait, and bruising. Group III includes physically abusive/resistive behavior, agitation, decreased sensation, hearing impaired, paralysis, contractures, need for mechanical lift, inability to balance, pitting edema, open lesions, purpuric lesions (3–4), and dry skin.

89. B: The Kennedy terminal ulcer phenomenon (first described by Karen Lou Kennedy-Evans) is the rapid development of pressure injury primarily in older adults with terminal illness and nearing death. The pressure injury occurs most often in the sacral area with an irregular or pear-shaped injury, although it can occur on heels, elbows, and posterior lower legs, and the area of ulceration may increase from stage 1 to stage 4 within a matter of hours. Terminal ulcers are usually not preventable.

90. D: If an immunocompromised patient develops a superficial infection on the left leg, spreading quickly with streaking, lymphedema, and clearly demarcated erythema and cellulitis, and the patient experience pain, moderate fever, and chills, these symptoms are consistent with erysipelas. Erysipelas is a bacillary infection that may result in systemic toxicity if untreated. Leukocytosis is generally present, and treatment is with oral or IV antibiotics. Erysipelas may occur with any break of the skin and is most commonly found on the legs or the face (associated with nasopharyngeal infection).

91. B: The appropriate initial response to a paraplegic patient who has developed a pressure injury is, "I'm so sorry this happened to you." Emotional support is important. Pressure injuries can occur with even the most conscientious patients, but patients often feel guilty or ashamed because of the negative attitude of healthcare providers and others. Questioning should be nonjudgmental: "When did you first notice that there was a pressure injury?" rather than "What happened?" (which suggests the patient did something to cause the pressure injury).

92. A: A skin barrier powder is used as an initial barrier on denuded skin to provide an adherent base for ointments, pastes, or solid skin adhesive barriers. The powder is sprinkled over the denuded area, and excess is removed before application of second barrier. The powder should be applied thinly because excess will impair adhesion of other barrier products, and it should not be used on intact skin, as it will not properly adhere. Skin barrier powders contain powder pectin, karaya, gelatine, carboxymethyl cellulose, or combinations. Skin barrier powders are frequently used with ostomy products when the skin has become weepy.

93. C: Integra, with a protective silicone outer layer over a collagen and chondroitin-6-sulfate layer, is FDA-approved for a wide variety of uses, including full-thickness or partial-thickness burns, pressure injuries, venous ulcers, diabetic ulcers, and surgical wounds, such as post-Moh's procedure. It is also used to resurface scars and keloids and for contracture release. Integra is usually meshed (1:1 ratio) to allow for drainage and penetration of antimicrobials. After application, Integra is secured with compression dressing or negative pressure.

94. B: During the inflammation phase, macrophages release growth factors, which attract fibroblasts to the wound. Fibroblasts are responsible for beginning angiogenesis and are critically important during the proliferation phase of healing, which usually begins at about day 3 after trauma. In addition to angiogenesis, fibroblasts initiate formation of collagen (type III) and initiate epithelialization, which begins from the basement membrane of the skin or from the wound edges if the basement membrane is compromised.

95. D: When educating a patient about preventing psoriasis, the patient should be advised to apply moisturizers to the skin because flareups are more likely to occur when the skin is dry. Therefore, flareups are more frequent when the weather is cold and dry. Patients should use a humidifier in the home in dry environments and should have some sun exposure because UV light is therapeutic. Patients may also need to avoid some medications if possible, including beta blockers, lithium, quinidine, and systemic corticosteroids.

96. A: Gauze dressings cause the most pain during dressing changes because they tend to adhere to the wound when dry. Even though wet-to-dry gauze dressings are frequently prescribed, they may result in trauma to the wound, damaging granulating tissue, and should be avoided in favor of dressing types that maintain a moist environment. The primary considerations when choosing a dressing type should be those that cause the least wound trauma and the least pain while promoting healing.

97. C: If an older patient has xerosis, tub baths should be limited to no more than 15 minutes to reduce drying of the skin, and the temperature should be tepid rather than hot. Showering is less drying. The patient should avoid vigorously scrubbing the skin and overuse of deodorant soaps, which alter the normal flora. Soaps should be pH balanced between 4.0 and 7.5, and the patient should be advised to apply moisturizers after the bath.

98. B: Contraction of the wound usually begins 5 days after injury. Contraction is the final step of the proliferation phase. Contraction is facilitated by fibroblasts (which produce and deposit extracellular proteins) and myofibroblasts, although it is not clear exactly how contraction occurs. Fibroblasts appear in the wound about 3 days after injury. Contraction is especially important in large wounds with tissue loss to help to provide wound closure and to reduce the time needed for healing.

99. A: Biofilms are large assemblages of microorganisms (planktonic bacteria) that adhere to surfaces. The biofilm may be comprised of multiple microorganisms that are able to exchange genetic material and communicate with each other and that are enclosed in an extracellular polymeric matrix. Risk factors for the development of biofilms include ischemia, wound necrosis, immunocompromise, and radiation therapy as well as inadequate nutrition. Biofilms tend to be antibiotic resistant and result in chronic inflammation.

100. C: If, following removal of a hydrocolloid wafer, the healthcare provider notes a malodorous gel-like substance on the skin side of the dressing, this likely indicates a normal finding from exudate. The exudate is absorbed by the gel-like substance of the wafer and combines to form a strong odor, which can be mistaken for signs of infection. Patients should be educated about the "gel and smell" of hydrocolloid dressings, especially if they are being taught to change their own dressings.

101. D: If a 54-year-old diabetic patient with heart disease developed a chronic (7 months duration) stage 4 coccygeal pressure injury following a stroke and the wound is large (7 x 5 x 1.5 cm) with copious exudate and signs of persistent infection, the best choice for wound care is to pack the wound with silver alginate and cover with bordered foam. Alginate absorbs exudate, and the silver has antimicrobial properties to help to combat the infection. The absorptive foam provides a warm moist environment to promote healing.

102. C: A partial thickness wound typically heals within about 14 days. Because the wound extends only into the dermis but does not go deep enough to severely damage the vessels, the skin is able to obtain the nutrition needed to repair itself fairly quickly. The initial bleeding activates hemostasis and provides some protection from bacteria. Vessels that are disrupted are sealed with a clot when coagulation takes place, and the clot later breaks down with fibrinolysis followed by repair during the proliferative stage.

103. A: Modified Wagner's Foot Ulcer Classification:

Grade 0	Pre-ulcerative but at risk. Healed ulcers or bony deformities may be present.
Grade 1	Superficial ulcer, extending into subcutaneous tissue; superficial infection with/without cellulitis.
Grade 2	Full-thickness ulcer to tendon or joint but no abscess or osteomyelitis.
Grade 3	Full-thickness ulcer may extend to bone with abscess, osteomyelitis, or sepsis of joint and may include deep plantar infections, abscesses, fascitis, or infections of tendon sheath.
Grade 4	Gangrene of the forefoot only, but the rest of foot is able to be salvaged.
Grade 5	Gangrene of entire foot, requiring amputation.

104. A: The best emollient to apply to the feet for a patient with peripheral neuropathy is petrolatum jelly as it has low water content and provides good moisturizing. Zinc oxide is used for barrier protection but is too thick for emollient purposes. Vicks VapoRub is used to soften calluses but not for routine foot care. Lotion has high water content and must be reapplied every few hours. Before application of petrolatum jelly, the feet should be washed (not soaked) with non-drying soap and dried thoroughly with clean cotton socks worn after application.

105. B: Lymphedema: Hard, non-pitting edema with skin thickening but no pigmentation. Edema usually includes the feet and toes and often occurs bilaterally. **Orthostatic edema:** Occurs with prolonged sitting and is soft and pitting but without skin thickening or pigmentation. It is always bilateral and includes edema of the foot. **Lipedema:** Bilateral fatty deposition in legs may mimic edema, but there is no pitting, skin thickening, or pigmentation and no edema of the foot. **Chronic venous insufficiency:** Edema is soft and pitting initially but may harden later. Skin thickening may occur about the ankle, and pigmentation changes are common. Edema often involves feet and may be bilateral.

106. A: If a patient has a wound infected with MRSA and is to receive treatment with ultraviolet light with a handheld device, the ultraviolet light should be held 1 inch from the wound with the device perpendicular to the wound. Ultraviolet light is usually used at wavelengths of 200–290 nm and is especially effective in killing bacteria, such as MRSA and other antibiotic resistant organisms. Ultraviolet light also stimulates granulation and wound debridement.

107. C: When using electrical stimulation (estim) for wound healing, most commonly high-voltage pulsed current, treatments are usually carried out 5–6 days per week for 45–60 minutes for each treatment. The electrodes are placed directly on the wound bed or adjacent to it. (Stocking and glove electrode garments are also available.) Estim can be used as a first-line treatment for wounds on the lower extremities, especially if circulation is impaired.

108. C: If a 5-year-old child has a series of bruises and lacerations in ovoid patterns suggesting bite injuries, which the parent states occurred when the child was playing with a toddler, and measurement of the intercanine distance is 3.2 cm, this likely indicates a bite from an adult as measurements over 3.0 cm are almost always from an adult. The appropriate authorities, such as Child Protective Services, should be notified of suspected child abuse.

109. A: These symptoms indicate grade I or mild envenomation, and 5 vials of antivenin are indicated. Grade II (moderate) envenomation, in which the pain and edema spread and systemic manifestations and mild coagulopathy occur, requires 5–15 vials, and grade III (severe) with severe systemic signs and coagulopathy, 15–20. Grade IV (life-threatening) requires 25 or more vials.

110. D: After applying becaplermin (a growth factor) gel (Regranex) to a diabetic ulcer, the wound should be covered with saline-moistened gauze. The gel is applied to about 1/16-inch thickness, and the dressing is left in place for about 12 hours and then removed, and the wound rinsed with saline or water in order to remove remaining gel. For the rest of the 24 hours, the wound should be covered with only a saline-moistened gauze.

Practice Test #2

1. To reduce risk of ulcerations, a patient with controlled bilateral peripheral pitting edema and brownish discoloration of skin around the ankles and anterior tibial areas should be advised to:

a. Wear sandals.
b. Wear compression stockings.
c. Use off-loading methods.
d. Avoid elevating feet above the heart.

2. TransCyte is indicated for treatment of:

a. Venous ulcers
b. Arterial ulcers
c. Surgical wounds
d. Burns (partial- to full-thickness)

3. The dietary requirement of protein to promote wound healing is:

a. 0.25–0.4 g/kg per day
b. 0.5–0.75 g/kg per day
c. 0.76–1.24 g/kg per day
d. 1.25–1.5 g/kg per day

4. According to CDC guidelines, which infection control precautions should be used when caring for a patient with osteomyelitis and a fistula infected with *Staphylococcus aureus*?

a. Standard and contact
b. Contact only
c. Standard only
d. Standard and droplet

5. An example of a wound that will probably undergo secondary healing is:

a. A split-thickness graft
b. An infected wound
c. An extensive contaminated dog bite wound
d. A clean laceration

6. When considering orthotics and shoe inserts for a patient with a neuropathic foot, which type of insert provides pressure relief?

a. Soft
b. Semi-soft
c. Rigid
d. Semi-rigid

7. Compression of tissue impairs circulation and can result in ischemia and pressure injury when the skin perfusion pressure falls to below:

a. 5–10 mmHg
b. 10–20 mmHg
c. 30–40 mmHg
d. 50–60 mmHg

8. The 5 basic elements of a skin assessment include (1) temperature, (2) color, (3) moisture, (4) integrity, and (5):

a. Pain
b. Turgor
c. Sensation
d. Edema

9. The best positioning to prevent pressure injuries is:

a. 30-degree tilt position, turning at least every 2 hours
b. 90-degree lateral side-lying position, turning every 2 hours
c. Prone position on alternating pressure mattress
d. Supine position on alternating pressure mattress

10. If the healthcare provider is using the NERDS mnemonic to identify a superficial infection, the "D" stands for:

a. Degeneration
b. Data
c. Dusky
d. Debris

11. Which is the best choice of barrier protection for intact skin to protect it from adhesive stripping and small amounts of exudate?

a. Skin sealant
b. Moister barrier ointment
c. Moisture barrier paste
d. Solid skin barrier

12. Chemical cauterization with silver nitrate is most commonly used on wounds to:

a. Debride ulcers.
b. Control bleeding.
c. Treat hypergranulation.
d. Decrease exudate.

13. In describing a wound, the term *slough* refers to:

a. Softening and irritation caused by skin contact with liquid
b. Bright pink or red granular appearing new tissue formed from capillary beds
c. Formation of healed tissue from epidermal cells over granulation
d. Soft viscous yellow layer of necrotic tissue that covers and adheres to the wound

14. When using Eutectic Mixture of Local Anesthetics (EMLA Cream) to relieve pain during dressing changes, what is the minimum duration of time the cream should be applied before beginning the dressing change?

a. 15 minutes
b. 30 minutes
c. 40 minutes
d. 60 minutes

15. If a wound is characterized by a defective matrix and cell debris that are impairing healing, which of the following is the correct intervention?

a. Negative pressure wound therapy
b. Moisture-balancing dressings
c. Antimicrobials
d. Debridement

16. With the TIME wound bed preparation approach, the "M" stands for:

a. Mechanical debridement
b. Measure of wound
c. Moisture balance
d. Maintenance of circulation

17. Venous ulcers are commonly:

a. Deep and circular
b. Superficial and irregular-shaped
c. Necrotic
d. Found on the toes and toe webs

18. The best action for a patient who is nearing death and has started to develop a pressure area on the sacral area but moans loudly and is resistive when the nurse assistant tries to turn him is to:

a. Turn the patient frequently to prevent further skin deterioration.
b. Allow the patient to lie undisturbed as much as possible.
c. Increase pain medication so that the patient can be turned.
d. Transfer the patient to a bed with an alternating pressure mattress.

19. What preparation is necessary for a patient who has a chronic leg ulcer covered with black eschar and is to have enzymatic debridement with collagenase?

a. Thoroughly drying the eschar and surrounding skin
b. Applying topical antibiotic
c. Scrubbing the wound with hexachlorophene
d. Crosshatching the upper layers of the eschar

20. Which of the following should the healthcare provider initially suspect if a wound has remained in the inflammation phase of healing for 10 days without progression and the surrounding skin has remained erythematous and edematous?

a. Infection
b. Inadequate protein intake
c. Secondary trauma
d. Immunosuppression

21. The type of wound likely to have the slowest rate of contraction is:

a. Linear
b. Square
c. Circular
d. Rectangular

22. Which diagnostic testing is most indicated for a patient who is a vegan and avoids all gluten-containing foods and legumes as well?

a. Prealbumin
b. BUN
c. Zinc level
d. Vitamin D level

23. Which of the following should be avoided when carrying out measures to prevent friction that may result in pressure injuries?

a. Talcum powder
b. Skin sealants
c. Cornstarch
d. Alcohol-based skin barrier

24. When evaluating a patient's nutritional status, what is the number of daily calories usually required for adequate wound healing?

a. 1000–1200 cal/day
b. 1500–3500 cal/day
c. 2000–4000 cal/day
d. 3000–6000 cal/day

25. When determining the severity level of a pressure injury using the Bates-Jensen Wound Assessment Tool (BWAT), a score of 42 indicates:

a. Minimal severity
b. Mild severity
c. Moderate severity
d. Critical severity

26. How would a wound be classified that healed as anticipated for the first week but then appeared to plateau and remained unchanged for the second and third weeks?

a. Chronic wound
b. Recalcitrant wound
c. Stunned wound
d. Acute wound

27. Which of the following treatments is initially indicated to relieve weepy, red, itchy atopic dermatitis?

a. Topical antihistamine
b. Wet aluminum acetate compresses
c. Hypoallergenic creams
d. Topical antibiotic

28. Which of the following complications may occur if a patient is placed in the prone position to relieve pressure on the hips and spine with the head positioned laterally?

a. Injury to the peroneal nerve as well as dislocation of the hip and stress on the lower back and pelvis
b. Increased intracranial pressure and increased intraocular pressure
c. Diaphragm displaced anteriorly by abdominal viscera resulting in decreased functional residual capacity, especially in the elderly
d. Decreased cerebral circulation and ocular damage

29. The most common site for venous ulcers is:

a. Medial malleolus
b. Lateral malleolus
c. Great toe
d. Medial aspect of knees

30. The primary reason for ambulating with an Unna boot is to:

a. Provide static support to the calf muscle pump.
b. Apply dynamic support to the calf muscle pump.
c. Apply continuous static compression to the lower leg.
d. Apply continuous dynamic support to the lower leg.

31. Which is the best support surface for a palliative care patient who cannot assume a variety of different positions without experiencing pain and exerting pressure on two existing pressure injuries, stages I and II?

a. Static flotation (water)
b. Foam
c. Alternating air mattress
d. High air loss (air-fluidized)

32. Which is the BEST dressing choice to absorb and contain the malodorous drainage from tumor necrosis resulting in a deep ulcerated area with a large amount of exudate?

a. Gauze
b. Open to air
c. Charcoal dressings
d. Foam

33. Which fistula management technique is probably best to prevent wound contamination from drainage for a large open post-surgical abdominal wound that has developed a fistula in the posterior aspect?

a. Simple pouching
b. Bridging
c. Saddlebagging
d. Troughing

34. The SAD (size, area, depth) grading classification is primarily used for:

a. Neuropathic ulcers
b. Pressure injuries
c. Venous ulcers
d. Arterial ulcers

35. Which of the following dressings provides moisture to dry wound beds, promotes autolysis of yellow slough, and softens black eschar?

a. Hydrocolloids
b. Alginate dressings
c. Transparent films
d. Hydrogels

36. Which of the following is the best method to assess the degree of undermining?

a. Visual inspection
b. Ultrasound
c. Palpation
d. Inserting a sterile swab

37. Which of the following lab values is indicative of dehydration?

a. BUN/creatinine ratio: 28:1
b. Urine specific gravity: 1.001
c. BUN 7: mg/dL
d. Serum osmolality: 290 mOsm/kg

38. At which stage in the healing of an incisional wound should a healing ridge be evident?

a. Inflammatory (days 1–4)
b. Proliferative (days 5–9)
c. Proliferative (days 10–14)
d. Proliferative to remodeling (day 15 onward)

39. When staging tissue damage from irradiation, how would moist, blistering tissue with epidermal tissue loss, serous drainage, and increased pain because of nerve exposure be classified?

a. Stage I
b. Stage II
c. Stage III
d. Stage IV

40. What is the best debridement choice for a pressure injury with hard dry black adherent eschar covering 75% of the wound?

a. Autolytic with transparent film dressing
b. Autolytic with hydrocolloid or hydrogel
c. Sharp
d. Enzymatic

41. Which class of compression stockings (such as Jobst or Therapress Duo) is indicated after edema is controlled to prevent venous ulcers for those at risk?

a. Class 1: 20–30 mmHg
b. Class 2: 30–40 mmHg
c. Class 3: 40–50 mmHg
d. Class 4: 50–60 mmHg

42. In a chronic wound, which phase of wound healing is generally prolonged?

a. Hemostasis
b. Inflammatory
c. Proliferative
d. Maturation

43. What is the best solution for applying negative pressure wound therapy (NPWT) to a large sacral wound that extends between the gluteal folds, preventing the adhesive dressing from sealing and resulting in a leak?

a. Cut foam large enough to fill the area where the leak occurs.
b. Discontinue NPT and institute a different kind of therapy.
c. Apply skin prep to the skin before applying adhesive.
d. Apply stoma paste to facilitate a seal.

44. When doing a pressure wound assessment using the Sussman Wound Healing tool, which of the following would be considered attributes that are "not good" for healing?

a. Fibroplasia
b. Contraction
c. Adherence
d. Erythema

45. Patient goals are developed from:

a. The problem list
b. Physician orders
c. The patient interview
d. Standardized goals associated with diagnosis

46. As circulation decreases in the lower extremities, what hair distribution changes occur?

a. No changes occur.
b. Hair is lost on toes only.
c. Hair is lost proximally.
d. Hair is lost distally.

47. Infrared thermography is especially useful for evaluating:

a. Extent of pressure injuries
b. Extent of infection
c. Risk of neuropathic ulcers
d. Phase of wound healing

48. Which of the following is generally the best method of realigning a 3 cm skin tear (Payne-Martin category I—Flap type) on the forearm on an 80-year-old patient?

a. Tissue glue
b. Sutures
c. Staples
d. Pressure dressing

49. During the monofilament test on the dorsum of the foot, the inability to perceive which force level is considered the threshold for loss of protective sensation?

a. 3.61
b. 4.17
c. 5.07
d. 6.10

50. What precaution is necessary when using pulsatile lavage with suction (PLWS) for mechanical debridement?

a. Allow only close family members in the room.
b. Use only if the patient's bed can be curtained off from others.
c. Disinfect the room prior to treatment.
d. Use only in a private room.

51. When conducting a pulse exam of the lower extremities, a pulse that is felt but diminished would be graded as:

a. 1+
b. 2+
c. 3+
d. 4+

52. At what angle should the Doppler probe be placed over the artery when assessing the brachial or ankle systolic pressure for the ABI?

a. 10 degrees
b. 30 degrees
c. 45 degrees
d. 90 degrees

53. The optimal sitting position to decrease risk of impaired perfusion is:

a. 95 degrees at hip and knee and 90–95 degrees at ankles
b. 90 degrees at hip, knees, and ankles
c. 90 degrees at hip, 95 degrees at knees and ankles
d. 90 degrees at hip and knees and 95 degrees at ankles

54. Sharp debridement would be recommended for which of the following?

a. Large pressure injury covered with moist necrotic tissue with evidence of increasing cellulitis
b. Large ischemic ulcer on ankle with evidence of cellulitis
c. Stable pressure area on heel covered by black eschar
d. Small pressure injury on right hip covered with yellow slough

55. Which type of wound usually produces the most exudate?

a. Arterial ulcer
b. Diabetic/neuropathic ulcer
c. Pressure injury
d. Venous ulcer

56. Which is the best debridement choice for a pressure injury with soft, stringy, adherent yellow slough covering 33% of the wound bed?

a. Enzymatic
b. Sharp
c. Autolytic with hydrocolloids or hydrogels
d. Autolytic with transparent film dressing

57. Apligraf, a biological skin substitute, is indicated for which of the following?

a. First-line treatment for infected venous ulcer
b. Diabetic ulcer (2-month duration) with muscle, tendon, capsule, or bone exposure
c. Diabetic ulcer (1-month duration) with no muscle, tendon, capsule, or bone exposure
d. Refractory venous leg ulcer (2-week duration)

58. For which of the following wounds would the use of a topical antiseptic be contraindicated?

a. Chronic venous ulcer
b. Second- and third-degree burns
c. Dog bite injury
d. Traumatic wound contaminated with debris

59. What is usually the appropriate pH to maintain in a wound and peri-wound tissue?

a. 4–5
b. 5–6
c. 6–7
d. 7–8

60. When using becaplermin gel to treat a diabetic ulcer, the gel should be left on the wound each day for:

a. 2 hours
b. 8 hours
c. 12 hours
d. 24 hours

61. What is the most likely treatment for a patient with venous insufficiency who develops pain and tenderness along the saphenous vein in the lower leg but without erythema or swelling?

a. Compression and NSAIDs
b. Warfarin or low molecular weight heparin
c. Bedrest and oral antibiotics
D. Compression and bedrest

62. Platelet-derived wound healing factor (PDWHF), such as AutoloGel, is derived from:

a. Pooled donor platelets
b. Single unrelated donor platelets
c. Single related donor platelets
d. Patient's own platelets

63. The correct procedure for obtaining a wound drainage specimen for aerobic culture is to:

a. Aspirate the wound drainage with a syringe without a needle.
b. Aspirate the wound drainage with a syringe with a needle.
c. Rotate a sterile swab in the drainage site.
d. Wipe the wound from side to side with a sterile swab.

64. Which of the following topical medications is effective against bacteria, viruses, and fungi?

a. Cadexomer iodine
b. Nystatin
c. Silver sulfadiazine
d. Metronidazole

65. Which of the following medications may contribute to bilateral peripheral edema?

a. Loop diuretics
b. Calcium channel blockers
c. Tricyclic antidepressants
d. Acetaminophen

66. What should be done prior to sharp debridement for a wound covered with dry eschar?

a. No further prep necessary
b. Mechanical debridement
c. Autolytic or enzymatic debridement
d. Pulsed lavage with suction

67. What is the most likely cause of a diabetic patient experiencing pain and diffuse swelling in the right foot, especially over the tarsometatarsal joint, with increased skin temperature of 5 degrees Fahrenheit?

a. Ischemia
b. Deep compartmental infection
c. Gout
d. Charcot arthropathy

68. An effective alternative to pressure dressing to treat hypertrophic scarring in a small area to which pressure cannot be easily applied is:

a. Massage
b. Silicone polymer gel
c. Tissue expanders
d. Surgical excision

69. The Vancouver Scar Scale, which is used to measure scar formation, assesses pigmentation and vascularity as well as:

a. Location and height
b. Location and deformity
c. Thickness and surface
d. Pliability and height

70. After acute surgery, the remodeling phase of wound healing of the incision usually lasts:

a. 2–4 months
b. 6–12 months
c. 1–2 years
d. 2–4 years

71. What is the NPIAP stage of a pressure injury that exhibits nonblanchable erythema and decreased skin temperature but intact skin?

a. Stage I
b. Stage II
c. Stage III
d. Stage IV

72. The best solution for a patient who has a small coccygeal pressure injury and can turn from side to side but bottoms out on her foam support surface and tends to slide down in bed is a:

a. Static air flotation device
b. Static water flotation device
c. Dynamic alternating air device
d. Low air loss device

73. For maintenance of skin to prevent drying and cracking, the choice that provides the longest duration of moisturizing is:

a. Lotions
b. Ointments
c. Creams
d. Oil baths

74. *Atrophie blanche* lesions are indicative of:

a. Venous insufficiency
b. Arterial insufficiency
c. Lipodermatosclerosis
d. Lymphedema

75. The best intervention for a diabetic patient with hammertoe and neuropathy to prevent ulceration is:

a. Tube foam
b. Sandal use instead of closed-toe shoes
c. Metatarsal pads
d. Crepe sole shoes

76. With the Sussman wound-healing protocol for high voltage pulsed current (HVPC) treatment, the duration and frequency of treatment for inflammation is:

a. 60 minutes, 5–7 times weekly for one week and then 3 times weekly for one week
b. 60 minutes, 5–7 times weekly
c. 60 minutes, 3–5 times weekly
d. 60 minutes, 3 times weekly

77. Which of the following can be used to stimulate erythema and restart the epithelialization phase of healing?

a. Vitamin C
b. Infrared radiation
c. Laser
d. Ultraviolet C light

78. What organism should be suspected if a burn wound develops increased thick greenish exudate with a foul musty fruity odor?

a. *Clostridioides difficile*
b. *Staphylococcus aureus*
c. *Streptococcus pyogenes*
d. *Pseudomonas aeruginosa*

79. What does it mean if a patient complains of increased pain during a pulsed short-wave diathermy treatment?

a. Inadequate heating
b. Unrelated to therapy
c. Expected response
d. Excessive heating

80. When evaluating edema, pitting to 4 mm that persists for 10–15 seconds would be classified on a 1–4 scale as:

a. 1+
b. 2+
c. 3+
d. 4+

81. In a wound, a biofilm may take on the appearance of:

a. Necrosis
b. Slough
c. Serosanguinous discharge
d. Purulent discharge

82. Which of the following is characteristic of moisture-associated and incontinence-associated dermatitis?

a. Presence of necrotic tissue
b. Lesions over bony prominences
c. Lesions in skin folds
d. Absence of pain/itching

83. If a patient has chronic pruritus and lesions from scratching, which of the following interventions should be part of the treatment plan?

a. Wear gloves at night.
b. Use silk or polyester sheets.
c. Use topical steroids daily.
d. Use negative reinforcement.

84. When applying an Unna boot over an open wound, the wound should be covered with a(n):

a. Foam dressing
b. Non-adherent dressing
c. Gauze dressing
d. Antibacterial ointment

85. With electrical stimulation (estim) using high-voltage pulsed current (HVPC), the negative electrode would be the active electrode if the wound is in the:

a. Hemostasis phase
b. Maturation phase
c. Proliferation phase
d. Inflammatory phase

86. Which of the following medications must be discontinued prior to treatment with hyperbaric oxygen?

a. Cisplatin
b. Methotrexate
c. Sulfathiazole
d. Fluoxetine

87. A patient with a small wound on the hand states he was bitten by a bat when he picked it up to remove it from his house. The most pressing need is:

a. Wound care
b. Antibiotic therapy
c. Rabies prophylaxis
d. Steroids

88. A fight-bite injury that occurs when a person strikes the teeth of another person with a clenched fist most commonly involves the dorsal surface of the:

a. Thumb (first)
b. Index finger (second)
c. Middle finger (third)
d. Ring finger (fourth)

89. Which of the following bacterial infections is most common after a cat bite?

a. *Staphylococcus aureus*
b. *Pasteurella multocida*
c. *Capnocytophaga canimorsus*
d. *Bartonella henselae*

90. When calculating the right dosage of becaplermin gel (Regranex), one should multiply the length and width of the wound in centimeters, and then divide by:

a. 2
b. 3
c. 4
d. 5

91. A patient stung by a stingray has excruciating pain at the site of injury. In addition to narcotics, which of the following interventions is indicated to relieve pain?

a. Topical steroid
b. Irrigation with vinegar
c. Ice packs
d. Heat immersion

92. To provide support for a scar, microporous tape should be applied:

a. Transversally at intermittent intervals along the scar
b. Longitudinally along the length of the scar
c. At right angles across the length of the scar
d. At right angles intermittently across the scar

93. Keloid scarring is generally caused by excess production of collagen type:

a. I
b. II
c. III
d. IV

94. Which of the following is a contraindication to the use of hydrocolloid dressings?

a. Leg ulcer
b. Surgical incision
c. Third-degree burn
d. Full-thickness wound

95. If a healthcare provider fails to provide adequate documentation regarding treatment outcomes, this may result in a:

a. Breach of duty
b. Claim of negligence
c. Loss of position
d. Disciplinary action

96. Which group of patients should be assessed for pressure injury risk?

a. All patients
b. Patients over 65 years
c. Patients with a history of pressure injuries
d. Patients with diabetes

97. Patients should be repositioned:

a. Routinely every 2 hours
b. Every 2–4 hours, depending on the patient's condition
c. Only if so ordered by the physician
d. As determined by the patient's condition and support surface utilized

98. According to CMS, in addition to daily wound monitoring, a thorough wound assessment should be carried out at least:

a. Daily
b. Weekly
c. Biweekly
d. Monthly

99. The primary purpose of photographing a wound is to:

a. Protect the organization from malpractice suits.
b. Facilitate assessment.
c. Show the progress of the wound.
d. Reduce the need for documentation.

100. If a patient scores 3 on the 1–4 scale in each of the 5 main categories (physical condition, mental condition, activity, mobility, and incontinence) of the Norton Pressure Ulcer Scale for a total score of 15, the patient's risk would be classified as:

a. Low
b. Medium
c. High
d. Very high

101. The best option for cleansing the perineal skin in patients at risk for incontinence-associated dermatitis is:

a. Water only
b. Mild soap and water
c. Disinfectant soap and water
d. Cleansing product pH balanced to that of the skin

102. An example of a humectant used in skin moisturizers is:

a. Petrolatum
b. Lanolin
c. Glycerin
d. Mineral oil

103. Which of the following skin conditions is characterized by a vesicular rash?

a. Erythema nodosum
b. Herpes zoster
c. Folliculitis
d. Candidiasis

104. The potency of topical corticosteroids may be increased by:

a. Air drying
b. Covering with a gauze dressing
c. Covering with a water-impermeable barrier
d. Applying heat to the area the steroid is applied to

105. Which of the following topical agents may be used to treat impetigo?

a. Clindamycin phosphate
b. Mupirocin
c. Dapsone
d. Erythromycin

106. Intertrigo is most likely to occur in patients that are:

a. Elderly
b. Diabetic
c. Obese
d. Malnourished

107. The most common cause of treatment-resistant acne vulgaris in adult females is:

a. Inadequate hygiene
b. Chronic MRSA infection
c. Polycystic ovary syndrome
d. Birth control pills

108. With cellulitis, blood testing usually shows leukocytosis with increased:

a. Neutrophils
b. Basophils
c. Lymphocytes
d. Monocytes

109. When conducting the history and physical exam of a new patient, the patient has multiple complaints and keeps interrupting the healthcare provider to discuss more issues, some major (abdominal pain) but some very minor (hangnail). The best response for the healthcare provider is to ask the patient to:

a. Answer questions briefly.
b. Help prioritize problems.
c. Explain in detail each complaint.
d. Only report major problems.

110. When utilizing the DIAPERS mnemonic to assess causes of acute urinary incontinence in a hospitalized patient with incontinence-associated dermatitis, the "D" refers to:

a. Dementia
b. Decreased sensation
c. Dehydration
d. Delirium

Answer Key and Explanations

1. B: Therapeutic compression stockings (class II, 30–40 mmHg) are used to prevent ulceration in those with varicose veins and stable venous insufficiency (indicated by brownish discoloration) after edema is controlled or with existing ulcers when edema recedes. Patients should also elevate feet when sitting. Therapy may include lying down and elevating affected limb above the heart for 1–2 hours two times daily and during the night. While everyone should stop smoking, it is more critical for those with peripheral arterial insufficiency.

2. D: TransCyte, which uses human neonatal fibroblasts on a nylon mesh protected by a silicone layer, is indicated for partial- or full-thickness burns as a temporary covering before autografting as well as for partial-thickness burns that will not require autografting. TransCyte must be applied to a clean wound base that has been freshly debrided. After application, TransCyte is secured with compression dressing or negative pressure and can last up to 100 days, although it must be removed if infection occurs or fluid begins to accumulate below the TransCyte.

3. D: Protein is critical for wound healing, and because metabolic rate increases in response to a wound, protein needs increase. The dietary requirement of protein for wound healing is 1.25–1.5 g/kg per day. A patient weighing 150 lb/68 kg would usually require about 60 g of protein daily but during wound healing, that need would increase to 85–102 g daily, so the patient would need to markedly increase their intake of high-protein foods or take dietary supplements. Meat, for example, contains only 7 g of protein per ounce.

4. A: Standard precautions—washing hands and wearing gloves and personal protective equipment (PPE) as needed for contact with bodily fluids—is used with all patients. However, patients with draining wounds, such as a fistula, should also have contact precautions, which require the use of PPE, including gown and gloves for all contact with the patient or the patient's immediate environment. The patient should be maintained in a private room or cohorted and should remain more than 3 feet away from other patients.

5. B: Secondary healing involves leaving the wound open to close through granulation and epithelialization. It is used with contaminated "dirty" or infected wounds to prevent abscess formation and allow drainage. Primary healing involves a wound that is surgically closed by suturing, flaps, or split or full-thickness grafts to completely cover the wound. It is used for surgeries or repair of wounds or lacerations, especially when the wound is essentially "clean." Tertiary healing involves first debriding the wound and allowing it to begin healing while open and then later closing the wound. It is used for contaminated wounds, such as severe animal bites, or wounds related to mixed trauma.

6. D: Semi-rigid inserts provide some cushioning as well as pressure relief. Soft inserts are used primarily for cushioning and to absorb shock. Rigid inserts, usually made from plastic, are used to maintain alignment or control abnormal motion. Accommodative inserts are inserts of multiple layers, reduced by half with compression. Shoes should be made of soft leather and should have enough depth to allow for inserts. Other modifications can include rocker soles, heel wrap, lateral flare, and mid-foot bolsters.

7. C: Compression of tissue impairs circulation and can result in ischemia and pressure injury when the skin perfusion pressure falls to below 30–40 mmHg. Normal skin perfusion pressure range is 50–100 mmHg. Skin perfusion pressure, which measures blood flow to a wound, may be assessed by applying sensors that detect oxygen about the wound in a normal room environment. The test may also be conducted in a hyperbaric chamber with the patient breathing 100% oxygen to determine if the oxygen content increases with hyperbaric oxygen treatment.

8. B: The 5 basic elements of a skin assessment include:

1. **Temperature**: Normally warm to the touch. Cool may indicate impaired circulation, and hot may indicate inflammation.
2. **Color**: Varies according to ethnicity, but pallor may indicate impaired circulation, while hyperpigmentation/hypopigmentation may indicate impaired circulation, disease or skin condition (altered melanin deposition).
3. **Moisture**: May vary from dry to moist, depending on general condition and skin disorders.
4. **Integrity**: Should be intact and free from open areas.
5. **Turgor**: Pinched skin should return to normal shape rapidly. Turgor may slow with dehydration and aging skin.

9. A: Because the 90-degree side-lying lateral position results in ischemia over bony prominences, patients should be positioned in the 30-degree tilt position as this causes less circulatory impairment. Goals for repositioning and a turning schedule of at least every 2 hours should be established for each individual, with documentation required. Devices, such as pillows or foam, should be used to correctly position patients so that bony prominences are protected and not in direct contact with each other. Pressure can occur even with alternating pressure mattresses.

10. D: NERDS mnemonic to identify a superficial infection:

- N: Non-healing wound is present.
- E: Exudate is present from the wound.
- R: Red and bleeding surface granulation tissue is evident.
- D: Debris includes yellow or black necrotic tissue on the surface of the wound.
- S: Smell or malodor is present from the wound.

11. A: Skin sealants are film-forming barriers composed of a polymer in a fast-drying solvent, applied every 1–4 days, depending on the product. When the sealant is applied to the skin, the solvent (often isopropyl alcohol) dissolves, leaving the transparent plasticized polymer barrier over the tissue. Skin sealant may be applied to intact or irritated tissue, although there may be some discomfort from the alcohol solvent with broken skin. Sealants can be used to protect skin from exudate, urine, stool, chemicals, and adhesive stripping. Sealants are applied with wipes, wands, or sprays.

12. C: Chemical cauterization with silver nitrate is sometimes used to treat hypergranulation. Cauterization uses heat to burn or sear abnormal cells in order to destroy them. Silver nitrate sticks are wet with water to activate and are then gently rolled for a short time over the tissue to be treated. The most common use for chemical cauterization in wounds or skin lesions is to control hypergranulation tissue that grows in wounds, especially about stomas. Hypergranulation tissue is often friable and bleeds easily. Treatment may be repeated 2 times daily for 1–4 days until excess tissue sloughs.

13. D: Slough is a soft viscous yellow layer of necrotic tissue that covers and adheres to the wound. **Granulation** is bright pink or red granular-appearing new tissue formed from capillary beds. **Eschar** is dark brown or black leathery necrotic tissue. **Epithelization** is the formation of healed tissue from epidermal cells over granulation. **Maceration** is the softening and irritation caused by contact with liquid. **Necrosis** is dead tissue. **Cellulitis** is inflammation of tissue, usually with edema and pronounced erythema.

14. B: Eutectic Mixture of Local Anesthetics (EMLA Cream) provides good pain control. The wound is first cleansed, and then the cream is applied thickly (1/4 inch), extending about 1/2 inch past the wound to the peri-wound tissue. The wound is then covered with plastic wrap, which is secured and left in place for a minimum of 30 minutes to reach its maximum effect. It may be applied for up to 60 minutes if necessary. The tissue should remain numb for about 1 hour after the plastic wrap is removed, allowing time for the wound to be cleansed, debrided, and/or redressed.

15. D: If a wound is characterized by a defective matrix and cell debris that are impairing healing, the correct intervention is debridement, which may be carried out episodically or continually, depending on the condition of the wound. Various methods of debridement may be utilized: autolytic, biological, sharp, mechanical, or surgical. The goal is to restore the wound base so that there is viable tissue that can begin the healing process.

16. C: TIME wound bed preparation approach:

- **T:** Tissue nonviable or deficient: Carry out debridement.
- **I:** Infection/inflammation: Administer topical/systemic antimicrobials, anti-inflammatories, and/or protease inhibitors.
- **M:** Moisture balance: Apply moisture-balancing dressings/therapy.
- **E:** Edge margin non-advancing or undermined: Utilize adjunctive therapies, bioengineered skin, debridement, and/or skin grafts.

17. B: Venous ulcers are typically superficial irregular ulcers on the medial or lateral malleolus and sometimes the anterior tibial area, causing varying degrees of pain. Surrounding skin often has brownish discoloration. Edema is moderate to severe. **Arterial ulcers** are painful, deep, circular, often necrotic ulcers found on toe tips, toe webs, heels or other pressure areas. There is often rubor on dependency but pallor on foot elevation, and skin is pale, shiny, and cool. Edema is minimal.

18. B: When a patient is nearing death, the most important consideration is comfort, even if this means that some routine patient care, such as turning the patient, must be set aside. The patient should be allowed to lie undisturbed as much as possible. Pain medication is usually decreased as a patient nears death, and increasing the medication may result in increased adverse effects. The process of transferring a patient to another bed may cause discomfort and distress.

19. D: Chemical debridement with enzymes is used for chronic wounds (burns, ulcers) with necrotic tissue and eschar. However, the enzymes (collagenase and papain/urea) require a moist environment, so the eschar must be crosshatched through the upper layers before the enzyme is administered. The pH must remain between 6 and 8 or the enzyme action is inactivated. Other causes of inactivation include hexachlorophene, Burrow's solution, and heavy metal ions. Collagenase is applied once daily, either directly to the wound for deep wounds or to gauze packing for shallow wounds.

20. A: When a wound remains in the inflammation phase of healing and does not progress to the proliferation phase, the most common reason is infection of the tissue. Inflammation may also be prolonged when necrotic tissue is present. The wound should be evaluated with culture and sensitivities to determine what interventions may be needed. Depending on the size of the wound and the degree of infection, an infected wound may be treated with IV, oral, or topical antibiotics.

21. C: Wound contraction occurs during phase III of healing, proliferation, when a ring of myofibroblasts develops beneath the skin, contracting the tissue. Circular wounds tend to contract slowly, while linear wounds (such as a surgical incision) contract rapidly, with square and rectangular wounds contracting at an intermediate rate. If contraction occurs too rapidly, it can result in excessive scarring, so contraction should be monitored and controlled, especially in areas such as the face, to avoid disfigurement, and hands, to avoid loss of mobility.

22. C: Because the patient's diet precludes animal protein as well as gluten-containing foods (such as wheat products) and legumes, the patient is at risk for zinc deficiency and should have zinc levels assessed. Supplementation should be provided, usually (usually 110–220 mg zinc gluconate or zinc sulfate TID). Zinc deficiency often coincides with vitamins A and D deficiency as well, so supplementation with these vitamins may be considered as well. Because the patient's diet is so restrictive, the patient should be evaluated for anorexia, which can also be an indication of zinc deficiency.

23. A: Friction by itself results only in damage to the epidermis and dermis, such as abrasions or denudement referred to as "sheet burn." Friction and pressure can combine, however, to form ulcers, so preventive measures are critical. Talcum powder may result in skin abrasion, so it should be avoided, although cornstarch can be applied to the skin or bed linens. Skin sealants and alcohol-based or non-alcohol-based skin barriers as well as skin lubricants may also provide protection from friction.

24. B: Adequate wound healing usually requires an intake of 1500–3500 calories per day, depending on the patient's age, size, and general condition. A lower caloric intake may restrict the protein necessary to promote the development of collagen and wound healing. If carbohydrate intake is too low, then the body may utilize protein for energy. Fats are necessary for construction of the cell membrane, and deficiency impairs healing. Patients need a well-balanced diet with vitamins and minerals. Vitamin C, vitamin A, iron, and copper are all important in the development of collagen.

25. D: A BWAT score of 42 indicates critical severity. BWAT comprises 13 categories: size, depth, edges, undermining, necrotic tissue type, necrotic tissue amount, exudate type, exudate amount, periwound skin color, peripheral tissue edema, peripheral tissue induration, granulation tissue, and epithelialization. Each category is scored from 1 to 5 with lower scores indicating lower severity. Scores are totaled to indicate severity:

- 13–20: minimal
- 21–30: mild
- 31–40: moderate
- 41–65: critical

26. C: A **stunned wound** appears to be healing well initially but then reaches a plateau and doesn't progress past that point of healing. An **acute wound** is from surgery or trauma and usually heals within an expected period of time without complications. A **chronic wound** persists more than 30 days and fails to progress. Some may never heal. A **recalcitrant wound** fails to follow a normal progression of healing and is difficult to manage because it fails to heal even with various treatments.

27. B: Wet aluminum acetate compresses are used to treat weepy lesions associated with atopic dermatitis. Atopic dermatitis (eczema) is a chronic inflammatory superficial skin disorder. It is related to allergies and associated with *xerosis*, which is dry skin with impaired barrier function. It is associated with dry or cold weather, central heating (which dries the air), and irritation caused by soaps and other skin cleaners. Skin is often red and itchy, and vesicles may develop, ooze, and crust. Skin may be rough, cracked, and scaly. Over time, skin may darken and thicken, and lichenification (markings from chronic scratching) may develop.

28. D: In the prone position, blood may pool in the extremities, and pressure on the abdomen may result in a decrease in BP, preload, and cardiac output. Respiratory effort increases, and lung compliance decreases. The head may be turned laterally, or if contraindicated because of arthritis or cerebrovascular disease, maintained in neutral position. Head positioned sharply to one side or the other may interfere with cerebral circulation. If head is turned laterally, then the dependent eye must be observed carefully for external compression that may cause ocular damage.

29. A: The medial malleolus is the most common site for venous ulcers because it is the distal point along the hydrostatic column of pressure and is distal to the calf pump and near the distal end of the lesser saphenous vein. Because of these factors, the medial malleolus is the point where venous pressure is the highest. However, ulcers may occur at any point between the knees and the ankle, so controlling edema and reducing venous hypertension is necessary as preventive measures.

30. A: The Unna boot is not in itself a compression device because the wrapping is applied firmly but with little tension. The patient must ambulate in order to gain benefit from the Unna boot, which becomes quite rigid after it is wrapped with elastic and provides static support. Because of the rigidity, as the person ambulates it forces the pressure from muscle contractions inward, and this pressure causes the one-way bicuspid valves of the calf muscle pump to open, forcing the blood upward and out of the area, reducing edema.

31. C: The alternating air mattress is a dynamic support surface and is especially useful for palliative care patients who cannot be moved easily without pain because it may assist with tissue perfusion even when patients are immobile. The support surface should be assessed with the patient in various positions for bottoming out by placing a flat hand beneath the patient's pressure points and ensuring there is at least an inch of support. Alternating air mattresses may result in moisture retention and heat accumulation.

32. C: While there are multiple ways to manage wounds with heavy exudate, in the context of malodorous wounds from tumor necrosis, charcoal dressings are most effective in both managing the exudate and absorbing the odor which can provide immense emotional relief to patients.

33. B: Bridging is a method to contain fistula drainage while protecting the wound from the exudate. A bridge is built with small pieces of barrier wafers, layering them until they are equal to the depth of the wound. This bridge is then adhered to the wound with barrier paste, and an ostomy pouch is then cut to fit the opening of the fistula. The ostomy pouch is applied to the intact skin on one side and the bridge on the other.

34. A: The SAD (size, area, depth) grading classification system, a modification of Wagner, is used for neuropathic ulcers. It includes evidence of sepsis, arteriopathy, and denervation as well. Ulcers are graded from **grade 0** (no evidence of pathology). **Grade 1** ulcers are $<10 \text{ mm}^2$ and extend into subcutaneous tissue. Exudate or superficial slough is present, and pulses are absent or diminished. Sensation is reduced. **Grade 2** ulcers are 10–20 mm^2 and can involve the tendons, joints, or periosteum. Cellulitis is present, but pulses may be absent. **Grade 3** ulcers are $>30 \text{ mm}^2$ and involve bones and joints. Osteomyelitis, Charcot's foot, and gangrene are evident.

35. D: Hydrogels are moisture-retentive, so they provide moisture to dry wound beds and promote autolysis of yellow slough and softening of black eschar. They are effective for partial- or full-thickness wounds with small amounts of exudate but are contraindicated with large amounts of exudate. They can be used with infected wounds. Hydrogels increase risk of yeast infections and may contribute to peri-wound maceration. Hydrogels are applied directly to the wound and covered with secondary dressings.

36. D: The best method to assess the degree of undermining is to insert a sterile swab into the undermined area, note the depth on the swab, and then measure it. Undermined areas may remain intact even though the tissue is damaged. In that case, the tissue should be palpated as it may feel spongy with the degree of undermining estimated. Undermining should be reported according to its relation to the open wound by reference to a clock face: "Undermining of 2.5 cm width extends from 1 o'clock to 2 o'clock."

37. A: Normal fluid requirements are 30 mL/kg of body weight or a minimum of 1,500 mL daily, although patients with draining wounds may require extra fluids.

- **BUN/creatinine ratio** >25:1 indicates dehydration, and <10:1 overhydration.
- **Urine specific gravity:** >1.028 g/mL indicates dehydration, and <1.002 g/mL overhydration.
- **BUN:** >35 mg/dL indicates dehydration, and <7 mg/dL overhydration.
- **Serum osmolality:** >303 mOsm/kg indicates dehydration, and >320 mOsm/kg overhydration
- **Serum sodium:** >145 mEq/L indicates dehydration, and <130 mEq/L overhydration.

38. B: Collagen deposit should create a palpable healing ridge along the incision during the phase of proliferation (days 5–9), and the ridge should be evident along the full length of the incision by day 9. It usually extends to about 1 cm on each side of the wound. If there is no evidence of the healing ridge by day 9, then the wound is at increased risk of dehiscence and infection. Sutures are usually removed from most wounds between days 5 and 9.

39. C: Staging of tissue damage from irradiation:

I	Inflammation results in increased edema and capillary permeability with erythema, itching, burning, and/or pain.
II	Skin is dry, itchy, and scaly, and epidermis begins to slough because of damage to basal epidermal cells and glands.
III	Epidermis continues to slough off, leaving skin moist and blistering with serous drainage and increased pain because nerves are exposed.
IV	Tissue changes include hair loss, atrophy, pigment changes, and ulcerations.

40. A: The best debridement choice for a pressure injury with hard dry black adherent eschar covering 75–100% of the wound is autolytic with transparent film dressing because the dressing traps fluid without absorbing it, more rapidly hydrating the eschar. The eschar should be crosshatched prior to application of the dressing to facilitate autolysis, and the circulation should be evaluated. Hydrogels and hydrocolloids may also be used; but, because they have absorptive properties, autolysis may take longer to be effective.

41. B: Class 2 compression stocking should be used after edema is controlled. Compression stockings are classified according to the degree of compression:

- Class 1: 20–30 mmHg, used for treatment of varicose veins
- Class 2: 30–40 mmHg used to prevent venous ulcers for those at risk
- Class 3: 40–50 mmHg used to treat refractory venous ulcers and lymphedema
- Class 4: 50–60 mmHg used to treat lymphedema

42. B: In a chronic wound, the inflammatory phase is generally prolonged because of the presence in the wound of neutrophils, which produce proinflammatory cytokines. As new tissue forms, it tends to become degraded through the action of proteinases. Most chronic wounds have full-thickness loss of tissue, resulting in the absence of the basement membrane to which epithelial cells generally attach, making epithelialization a more complex and lengthy process. Chronic wounds are also susceptible to the growth of biofilms, which retard healing.

43. D: NPWT is often applied to areas where the tissue is discontinuous or skin folds interfere with adherence of the adhesive dressing, so the best solution is to apply stoma paste to the area where the leak is occurring to create a bridge to which to apply the clear adhesive dressing. The foam should be cut to fit the wound, so that when negative pressure is applied (tested by pressing down with a finger), the foam does not overlap the wound, as this may result in maceration of the tissue.

44. D: SWHT was developed to monitor healing of pressure wounds. Part I assesses 5 tissue attributes classified as "not good" for healing: hemorrhage, maceration, undermining, erythema, and necrosis. It also assesses 5 tissue attributes that are "good" for healing: adherence, granulation, contraction, sustained contraction, and epithelialization. Part II assesses wound depth and tunneling/undermining. Additional attributes include describing the location of the wound and the healing phase, described as chronic, acute, or absent.

45. A: Goals are developed from the problem list that is generated as part of the plan of care, based on patient interview, history, physical exam, and medical records. Goals should be specifically related to the problem, measurable by some method, and attainable. Goals may focus on three areas:

- Resolution: "Pulse rates will not exceed 90 at rest."
- Preventing deterioration or further complications: "Patient will remain at current weight."
- Palliation/patient comfort: "Patient will not experience break-through pain."

46. D: As circulation decreases in the lower extremities, hair distribution is lost distally, so assessing hair distribution is one measure to evaluate impaired circulation. Because hair follicles provide epidermal cells that are important for resurfacing of partial-thickness wounds, the absence of hair can negatively affect healing, especially in areas where hair has been lost. The hair on the great toes should be assessed because lack of hair (if not shaven) indicates circulatory impairment. The hair distribution on the leg should be evaluated to determine the most distal area of hair growth.

47. C: Infrared thermography is especially useful for evaluating the risk of neuropathic ulcers. While fever strips are often used to evaluate increased temperature about a wound, they are not as sensitive to measure subtle changes. People at risk for neuropathic ulcers often have an impaired immune system, so the usual signs of inflammation (erythema at the site of damaged tissue) may not be evident, but the temperature of the area may be increased and detectable by infrared thermography.

48. A: Because Payne-Martin category I injuries align well, tissue glue is probably the best choice because it minimizes drainage and keeps the flap securely in place. Mature skin is generally more friable than younger skin, so sutures and/or staples may cause more trauma and should be avoided if possible. A pressure dressing alone may not provide adequate alignment because dressings can shift. Also, dressings may adhere to the wound, causing increased trauma during removal. When adhesive strips are used, they must be spaced to allow for drainage.

49. C: The force level considered the threshold for loss of protective sensation with the monofilament test on the dorsum of the foot is 5.07, while an inability to perceive a force level of 4.56 on the plantar surface of the foot indicates loss of protective sensation. An inability to perceive force level of 3.61 is considered within normal parameters, but those who cannot perceive 5.07 force level are at increased risk because their ability to use protective sensations is limited.

50. D: Because microorganisms can become aerosolized during treatment with PLWS, the patient must be treated in a private room with the door closed to ensure contamination does not spread; curtaining off the patient is not adequate. There should be no visitors or family present during treatment, and any other open wounds, ports, IV's or other tubes on the patient should be covered. The nurse should wear appropriate PPE. The room must be thoroughly disinfected after treatment.

51. A: A pulse that is felt but diminished is graded as 1+. The pulse exam for vascular evaluation of the lower extremities should be conducted bilaterally with the femoral, popliteal, dorsalis, pedis, and posterior tibial artery pulses. The popliteal pulse is most easily assessed with the patient in the prone position. Pulses are graded from 0 to 4+:

- 0: No pulse palpable.
- 1+: Pulse is weak and difficult to palpate.
- 2+: Pulse is normal.
- 3+: Pulse is full.
- 4+: Pulse is abnormally bounding, aneurysmal.

52. C: ABI procedure (do bilaterally and use higher readings):

1. Apply blood pressure cuff to one arm, palpate brachial pulse, and place conductivity gel over artery.
2. Place tip of a Doppler device at a 45-degree angle into gel at brachial artery, and listen for pulse sound.
3. Inflate cuff until pulse sound ceases, and then inflate 20 mmHg above that point.
4. Release air and listen for return of pulse sound for brachial systolic pressure.
5. Repeat same procedure on each ankle with cuff applied above the malleoli and gel over the posterior tibial pulse for ankle systolic pressure.
6. Divide ankle systolic pressure by brachial systolic pressure to obtain the ABI.

53. A: The optimal sitting position is 95 degrees at hip and knees and 90–95 degrees at the ankles. The 95-degree angle at the hip and knees allows the patient to sit upright while interfering less with perfusion than when a patient is sitting at 90 degrees. Patients should be carefully evaluated for range of motion and ability to sit in an upright position as modifications must be made for those with limited range of motion. Feet should be supported when patients are in sitting position.

54. A: Sharp debridement would be recommended for the large pressure injury covered with moist necrotic tissue with evidence of cellulitis as it may convert the wound from necrotic to acute and clean, promoting healing. Sharp debridement may be done in conjunction with other methods, such as enzymatic, mechanic, or autolytic debridement, to soften eschar. Ischemic ulcers should not undergo sharp debridement, and stable pressure areas covered by black eschar on the heels are usually left intact as the eschar provides some protection. Small pressure injuries with yellow slough may be treated with other forms of debridement.

55. D: Because venous wounds are usually associated with peripheral edema, they tend to produce the most exudate throughout the healing process, so providing gradient compression to reduce edema is an important aspect of treatment. Venous wounds may be covered with yellow fibrinous material that can appear to be exudate. Arterial wounds tend to be dry or to have slight exudate. Neuropathic wounds usually have minimal serous or serosanguineous exudate. Pressure injuries have varying amounts of exudate, depending on the wound characteristics.

56. C: Because slough provides a moist environment, the best choice for debridement is autolytic with hydrocolloids or hydrogels because they have absorptive properties to contain exudate while maintaining the moist environment to facilitate autolysis. Enzymatic debridement may also be considered, but the agent chosen must be effective against collagen and protein, and the surrounding skin must be protected from the enzyme and exudate, or maceration may occur. In some cases, sharp debridement may be done, often in conjunction with autolytic debridement.

57. C: Apligraf is FDA-approved for diabetic ulcers of more than 2 weeks duration with no muscle, tendon, capsule, or bone exposure as well as venous leg ulcers that have been refractory to other treatments and persisted for more than a month. Apligraf is composed of two layers. The epidermal layer is from neonatal keratinocytes (from neonatal foreskin), and the dermal layer is from bovine collagen seeded with neonatal fibroblasts. Apligraf should not be used in infected wounds or with necrosis.

58. A: Topical antiseptics are generally contraindicated in the treatment of chronic wounds, such as a venous ulcer, as they have little value and may cause injury to tissue. Topical antiseptics only affect bacteria on the wound surface but cannot reach infected tissue, so wound infection is better treated with systemic antibiotics. Topical antiseptics, however, are used with acute wounds, such as dog bites and other traumatic contaminated wounds, to prevent infection and may be indicated with patients who are immunocompromised. They are also routinely used with burns because necrotic tissue can lead to infection.

59. B: Wounds and peri-wound tissue should be maintained with an acid pH of 5–6, so most skin cleansers, which tend to be alkaline, should be avoided in favor of irrigating the wound with water or normal saline. Any cleansing materials should be used at body temperature (lukewarm) as cold solutions may interfere with wound perfusion. Direct contact with granulating tissue should be minimal. Skin or wound cleansers with surfactant properties, along with irrigants, may help to remove debris.

60. C: Becaplermin (Regranex Gel) is a growth factor used to promote wound healing of diabetic/neuropathic ulcers that extend into or beyond the subcutaneous tissue but have adequate perfusion. The wound is coated with 1/16th inch of gel and covered with gauze moistened with NS, which is left in place for 12 hours. Then the dressing is removed, and the wound is irrigated with NS and covered with gauze moistened with NS for the next 12 hours. This procedure is repeated daily.

61. A: Pain and tenderness along the saphenous vein in the lower leg is usually associated with superficial phlebitis and treated with compression and NSAIDs and continued ambulation as risk for development of DVT is low. However, if erythema, swelling, and marked pain occur, this may indicate DVT, which should be confirmed with Doppler. DVT may be treated with anticoagulation (warfarin, heparin) or thrombolysis, although thrombolysis increases risk of hemorrhage or stroke. The affected leg is elevated with use of a compression device to reduce swelling.

62. D: Platelet-derived wound healing factor (PDWHF), such as AutoloGel, is derived from the patient's own platelets, so it is prepared individually. It is used to initiate coagulation and provide growth factors to improve and hasten healing. The gel is applied topically and left in place for 5 days, after which an alternative dressing is applied for 7 days, and then the cycle is repeated until wound healing occurs. AutoloGel has been used effectively to treat diabetic neuropathic ulcers involving deep structures, such as tendons and fascia.

63. C: Aerobic cultures are for bacteria that grow when exposed to air, so the appropriate method is to remove a sterile swab from a culture tube, rotate it gently in an area of drainage in the wound, return the swab to the culture tube, crush the ampule containing medium, and push the swab into the medium as this helps to keep the bacteria viable until the sample can be analyzed. Anaerobic cultures are taken from deeper in the wound and aspirated with a syringe without a needle.

64. A: Cadexomer iodine prepared as a paste, powder or ointment is effective against a broad range of bacteria (MRSA, *Staph, Strep, Pseudomonas)* as well as viruses and fungi and promotes healing. **Nystatin** is an antifungal agent and may be used prophylactically or to control a fungal infection. **Silver sulfadiazine** is incorporated into a number of dressings for antibacterial action, but it is commonly used to prevent wound sepsis and reduce bacterial load in burns. **Metronidazole**, in gel, cream, or lotion, is effective against bacteria, including MRSA.

65. B: A number of medications can contribute to peripheral edema, especially calcium channel blockers and other antihypertensives (hydralazine, reserpine, BBs, and clonidine) and corticosteroids, as well as hormones (estrogen, testosterone, progesterone), NSAIDS, Cox-2 inhibitors, and MOAIs. The patient's medications should be carefully reviewed as some, such as corticosteroids, as well as causing edema, may also impair healing. Drugs that interfere with cell division, such as chemotherapeutic and immunosuppressive agents, and those that inhibit clotting, such as anticoagulants, also can impair healing.

66. C: Prior to debriding a wound covered with dry eschar, the eschar should be softened with autolytic or enzymatic debridement because a moist necrotic wound is easier to debride than a dry one, especially if the eschar is firmly adhered to the wound. Additionally, sharp debridement on wounds covered with dry eschar is contraindicated without a vascular consultation to assess circulation. The eschar should be crosshatched prior to autolytic or enzymatic debridement. A combination of autolytic/enzymatic debridement and sequential sharp debridement is often the most effective.

67. D: Charcot arthropathy may be atrophic or hypertrophic (most common) and can cause joint deformities and fractures. Typical indications include pain and swelling of the foot along with increased skin temperature of at least 4 degrees F. Pain may be less severe than expected because of loss of protective sensation. Charcot arthropathy may occur with plantar ulcers or with intact skin and may be misdiagnosed as osteomyelitis. Treatment includes offloading, such as with a total contact cast.

68. B: Silicone polymer gel (supplied in sheets or pads of various sizes and shapes) is placed directly over a maturing scar to treat hypertrophy. Silicone is usually used on small scarring areas or areas where pressure cannot be easily applied. Some people may develop a rash from the silicone, but this usually clears easily if the silicone treatment is withheld for a few days, after which it may be reapplied. Skin breakdown rarely occurs unless a rash occurs and the silicone is left in place.

69. D: The Vancouver Scar Scale, which is used to measure scar formation, assesses pigmentation and vascularity as well as pliability and height, with each parameter scored from 0 (normal) to 3–5 (severe), with a higher score indicating a worse scar:

- Pigmentation ranges from normal to hypopigmentation to hyperpigmentation.
- Vascularity ranges from normal to pink, red, and purple.
- Pliability ranges from normal to supple, yielding firm, banding and contracture.
- Height ranges from flat to raised >2mm, raised <5 mm and raised >5mm.

70. C: The remodeling phase of an acute surgical incision may persist for 1–2 years. Usually, the incisional color lightens from red to white over the course of the first year, while the tensile strength gradually increases to about 80% of normal during the same time. During the remodeling phase, it's important for the patient to avoid excessive force or tension on the wound as this may interfere with healing or result in excessive scarring.

71. A: This is a stage I pressure injury. NPIAP stages:

- Stage I: Skin intact with localized non-blanching erythema, decreased skin temperature.
- Stage II: Abrasion, blister, or slightly depressed area with red/pink wound bed but no slough. Partial thickness superficial skin loss.
- Stage III: Deep full-thickness ulceration that exposes subcutaneous tissue with possible presence of slough, tunneling and undermining but without visibility of underlying muscle, tendon, or bone.
- Stage IV: Deep full-thickness ulceration with extensive damage, necrosis of tissue extending to muscle, bone, tendons, or joints.
- Unstageable: Extent of slough/eschar render ulcer unstageable before debridement.
- Suspected deep tissue injury: Purple/reddish discoloration and boggy, mushy or firm tissue caused by pressure and/or shear.

72. C: Since bottoming out means that there is less than an inch of support and the patient tends to slide down in bed, which can result in shear, the best choice for this patient is to switch to a dynamic alternating air device, which provides increased support as well as shear and pressure reduction. While this type of surface is more expensive than static devices, it is more moderately priced than low air loss or high air loss devices.

73. B: Ointments, usually lanolin or petrolatum-based, have the lowest water content and provides the longest duration of moisturizing and usually must be reapplied once or twice daily. Many oils and lotions are used to increase hydration of the skin. These can include oil baths, which have a minimal effect on hydration but do increase the skin-surface lipids. Lotions have high water content and must be applied 5–6 times daily, while creams, which contain water and oil, require application about 4 times daily.

74. A: *Atropie blanche* lesions are smooth white avascular sclerotic skin plaques that occur in about one-third of patients with lower extremity venous disease. They are associated with pain while standing and at rest. The lesions are usually associated with torturous vessels and hemosiderin staining on the ankles or foot, other indications of venous disease. They may appear similar to scarring from healed ulcers but actually have a high risk for deteriorating into ulcer formation.

75. A: Hammertoes, corns, and claw toes and small lesions on the toes should be cushioned with tube foam or lamb's wool. Tube foam can be cut to fit and separates the toes to allow airflow and prevent skin irritation and pressure from the shoe. Sandals should be avoided by diabetic patients because they leave part of the foot exposed and at risk of trauma. Metatarsal pads relieve pressure on metatarsal heads, and crepe sole shoes provide support for the plantar surface of the foot.

76. B: Sussman's wound healing protocol for HVPC for treatment of inflammation requires 60-minute treatments 5–7 days per week. The polarity is set at negative, the pulse rate frequency at 30 pps, and the intensity at 100–150 V. Edema protocol requires negative polarity, pulse rate frequency of 30–50 pps, intensity of ≤150 with 60-minute treatments 5–7 times a week for one week and then 3 times a week for one week.

77. D: Ultraviolet C light, which has bacteriocidal properties, can be used to produce a second-degree burn, which causes an inflammatory response that may restart epithelialization in a wound with delayed healing. Other options to promote epithelialization include the use of topical or oral vitamin A and application of electrical stimulation. Topical vitamin A may promote macrophage activity. Some studies have indicated that statins, used to treat high cholesterol, also stimulate epithelialization and have a beneficial effect on healing.

78. D: *Pseudomonas aeruginosa,* characterized by thick green exudate and foul musty fruity odor, is a Gram-negative aerobic bacillus that favors moist conditions. *P. aeruginosa* is encapsulated, providing protection from antibodies, and produces toxins, enzymes, cytotoxins, and hemolysins that resist phagocytosis and destroy cells of the host. *P. aeruginosa* is an opportunistic infection, invading compromised tissue. It can cause severe infections of virtually all systems and is especially dangerous for those with severe burns or with immunosuppression. Additionally, *P. aeruginosa* is resistant to many common antibiotics, and some strains have proven resistant to all antimicrobials.

79. D: Patients experience pain with excessive heating from pulsed short-wave diathermy, which is used to increase blood flow, oxygenation, and metabolic rate and promote healing. It is also used to relieve pain and edema, so patients should be monitored closely; if pain increases or occurs, the power level should be reduced or air space increased. Care must be taken to avoid any contact with metals or synthetic materials, which increases risk of burns. Electronic devices (watches, hearing aids) should be removed prior to treatment.

80. B: This edema is 2+. Edema is usually checked by pressing the index finger into the tissue on top of each foot, behind the medial malleolus, and over the shin, starting distally and moving proximally to the highest level of edema, comparing both legs. The grading scale is as follows:

- 1+: slight pitting to about 2 mm (persists 10–15 seconds)
- 2+: moderate pitting to about 4 mm (persists 10–15 seconds)
- 3+: moderate-severe pitting to about 6 mm (persists >1 minute)
- 4+: severe pitting to 8 mm or more (persists 2–5 minutes)

81. B: In a wound, a biofilm may take on the appearance of slough, so it may be a challenge to differentiate the two, although a biofilm tends to have a shinier and more gel-like appearance from the extracellular polymeric matrix that encloses the biofilm. In fact, the biofilm causes a chronic inflammation that results in increased permeability of vessels and increased exudate, leading to the production of slough, so the presence of slough may be an indication that a biofilm is present. Treatment includes debridement and dressings and topical antibiotics to prevent reformation of the biofilm.

82. C: Moisture-associated and incontinence-associated dermatitis is characterized by lesions in skin folds (such as the labia, between the buttocks, and under and around the scrotum) rather than over bony prominences. The inflamed tissue tends to be red and diffuse rather than circumscribed and red to purple as in pressure injuries. The dermatitis may vary from intact but irritated skin to partial-thickness wounds. Necrotic tissue is not present although patients may complain of pain and itching.

83. A: If a patient has chronic pruritus and lesions from scratching, the intervention that should be part of the treatment plan is to wear gloves at night because patients often experience increased itching and scratching during the night. The patient should also keep the nails short and should use cotton sheets and avoid wearing clothing that may increase the pruritus, such as rough-textured or woolen clothing. Topical emollients may provide some relief, but chronic use of topical steroids should be avoided.

84. B: When applying an Unna boot over an open wound, the wound should be covered with a non-adherent dressing to prevent traumatic injury to the healing tissue when the Unna boot is removed. Unna boots are indicated for wounds that are slow healing and are usually left in place for 3–7 days and serve to protect the wound and to promote healing. The wound should be carefully assessed at each change.

85. D: With electrical stimulation (estim) using high-voltage pulsed current (HVPC), the negative electrode would be the active electrode if the wound is in the inflammatory phase. One electrode is the active one (negative or positive), and the other is the dispersive electrode. The electrodes attract particular cells. The negative electrode typically attracts neutrophils, fibroblasts, and lymphocytes, making it effective for infected wounds. The positive electrode would be the active electrode on the wound if the wound is clean and in the proliferation phase. The positive electrode attracts macrophages and is effective in necrotic wounds.

86. A: Cisplatin and Sulfamylon must be discontinued prior to treatment with hyperbaric oxygen because the combination of the drug and the therapy impairs wound healing. Other drugs that must be discontinued include bleomycin (which can lead to interstitial pneumonitis), disulfiram (which can lead to oxygen toxicity), and doxorubicin (which can lead to oxygen toxicity). Both bleomycin and cisplatin must be discontinued for an extended time period before beginning hyperbaric oxygen therapy.

87. C: If a patient with a small wound on the hand states he was bitten by a bat when he picked it up to remove it from his house, the most pressing need is rabies prophylaxis because bats have a high rate of rabies infection. A bat that is able to be picked up is probably ill, and that increases the risk. All bites from a bat, even tiny wounds, must be treated with post-exposure prophylaxis before the onset of any symptoms in order to be effective.

88. C: A fight-bite injury that occurs when a person strikes the teeth of another person with a clenched fist most commonly involves the dorsal surface of the middle (third) finger. Because the fist is clenched when the injury occurs, when the person straightens the fingers, bacteria that was inoculated into the wound spreads proximally with the extensor tendons. This type of wound is difficult to irrigate and is at high risk of infection, so antibiotic prophylaxis is indicated.

89. B: Up to 80% of infections after a cat bite result from *Pasteurella multocida,* with signs of infection evident within 2–12 hours. Infection begins with local inflammation but can spread to bones and joints if bacteria were inoculated deeply and systemically, resulting in multiple disorders, including pneumonia, meningitis, endocarditis, pericarditis, peritonitis, hepatosplenic abscesses, conjunctivitis, pyelonephritis, cervicitis, and epididymitis. Treatment is with broad-spectrum antibiotics.

90. C: The dosage for becaplermin gel (Regranex), a growth factor, is calculated in centimeters by multiplying the greatest length and greatest width of the wound and dividing by 4. Thus, if the wound were 6 cm long and 4 cm wide, the dosage would be calculated as: 6 X 4/4 = 24/4 = 6 cm of gel. The dosage should be recalculated at least once a week or as the ulcer changes in size.

91. D: If a patient stung by a stingray has excruciating pain at the site of injury, in addition to narcotics, the intervention that is indicated to relieve pain is heat immersion, which helps to deactivate the venom. The wound should be immersed in water (110–115 °F/43.3–46 °C) for 30–90 minutes at a time and may be repeated up to 2 hours. A local anesthetic, such as lidocaine or bupivacaine, may be administered if the patient does not have adequate relief from heat immersion.

92. B: To provide support for a scar, microporous tape should be applied longitudinally along the entire length of the scar and left in place until it loosens on its own after several days before replacement. Stripping the tape may cause inflammation that worsens the scar. The tape should not be applied at right angles. Scar support is especially important in areas where vector forces pull at the wound, such as in areas of movement.

93. A: Keloid scarring is generally caused by excess production of collagen type I, which is found in the skin. There is a genetic component to keloid scarring, which involves fibrous tissue that develops about a wound. The keloid scar may develop over a period of about 3 months and can be larger than the original wound, having the appearance of tumors at times. Keloid scarring is most common in patients with darkener skin tones, such as African Americans, Asians, and Latinos.

94. C: A contraindication for the use of hydrocolloid dressing is a third-degree burn, although they may be used in small partial-thickness burns, especially in the later stages of healing. Hydrocolloid dressings are generally contraindicated for infected wounds and those with tunneling as well as dry wounds and those with heavy exudate. Hydrocolloid dressings should also be avoided if the periwound tissue is very fragile as they may result in further skin breakdown when removed.

95. B: If a healthcare provider fails to provide adequate documentation regarding treatment outcomes, this may result in a claim of negligence. The medical record is a legal document, so information that is missing from the record may be used as the basis for claims that care was not provided or was inadequate. The medical record is the primary means of communication among different healthcare providers (physicians, nurses, physical therapists, other therapists) as most members of the team may be absent from oral reports.

96. A: All patients should be routinely assessed for pressure injury risk, even though some groups, such as those over 65, those with a history of pressure injuries, and those with diabetes, may be at increased risk. Focusing only on limited groups may result in missing other patients who may develop pressure injuries. Various risk scales, such as Braden or Norton, may be utilized and can help to determine the care needs of the patient.

97. D: Patients should be repositioned according to the patient's condition and the support surface utilized rather than on a routine "q 2 hr" basis, which has been the standard for many years. Some patients may require more frequent turning, and others may be able to turn independently. Support surfaces that redistribute pressure may allow patients to be left in place for longer periods. The patient's risk for pressure injuries should be part of the consideration for repositioning.

98. B: According to CMS, in addition to daily wound monitoring, a thorough wound assessment should be carried out at least weekly. The wound assessment should ideally be carried out by a wound care specialist. Small changes may be overlooked in daily monitoring but may be more evident over a more extended period of time. Documentation of wound condition should be done in a consistent manner so that all healthcare providers are following the same protocol.

99. C: The primary purpose of photographing a wound is to show the progress of the wound, so a series of photographs taken at regular intervals is more valuable than photographs simply taken on admission or occasionally. Photography should not be used as a substitute for documentation, and each photograph should be accompanied by a written description of the wound. Healthcare organizations may have various protocols for photography, although noninvasive photography of wounds does not generally require written consent.

100. B: If a patient score 3 on a 1–4 scale in each of the 5 main categories (physical condition, mental condition, activity, mobility, and incontinence) of the Norton Pressure Ulcer Scale for a total score of 15, the patient's risk would be classified as medium:

- 19–20: low risk
- 14–18: medium risk
- 10–14: high risk
- 5–9: very high risk

The Norton Pressure Ulcer Scale has been used since 1962 and was developed in England. The Braden Scale is more frequently used because it evaluates more factors, but the Norton Scale is still often used because of its simplicity.

101. D: The best option for cleansing the perineal skin in patients at risk for incontinence-associated dermatitis is a cleaning product pH balanced to that of the skin. No rinse cleansers should be utilized, and scrubbing should be avoided. Soap should also be avoided as it may increase irritation. Additionally, moisturizers and skin barriers (such as zinc oxide) should be applied to protect the skin. Antifungal products may be necessary as well because the warmth and dampness of incontinence encourages the growth of fungal infections.

102. C: An example of a humectant used in skin moisturizers is glycerin. Humectants are included to promote water retention in the stratum corneum. Other humectants commonly used include urea, propylene glycol, proteins, and urea. Other ingredients in moisturizers include occlusives, which provide protection to decrease water loss to the environment, and emollients, which aid in hydration of the stratum corneum. Occlusives include palm kernel, castor oil, carnauba wax, allantoin and cocoa butter. Emollients include mineral oil, cocoa butter, lanolin, paraffin, and shea butter.

103. B: Skin conditions characterized by a vesicular rash include herpes zoster as well as herpes simplex. Vesicles have the appearance of blisters but are small, typically 5–10 mm in diameter, and result from fluid under the epidermis. If the lesions are 0.5 cm or larger, they are referred to as bullae. Other causes of vesicular rash include chicken pox (varicella), acute contact dermatitis, pompholyx, scabies, and some rashes associated with drugs.

104. C: The potency of topical corticosteroids may be increased by covering with a water-impermeable barrier, such as plastic wrap or gloves (if on the hands). The covering should be kept in place for at least 4 hours. Alternately, wet wraps may be used for large areas, such as having the patient wear damp pajamas covered with dry pajamas. Topical steroids have very little systemic absorption, so they have fewer adverse effects than oral steroids. Ointments are more potent than creams.

105. B: Mupirocin (Bactroban) is a topical agent that may be used to treat impetigo. Mupirocin is available in ointment or cream and is usually applied 3 times daily. If the patient has nasal colonization of *Staphylococcus aureus* or MRSA, mupirocin may be applied in the nares twice daily for 5 days to reduce carriage. Mupirocin may also be used to treat folliculitis and furunculosis. Adverse effects may include mild burning or stinging. Extensive use may also result in *Clostridioides difficile*-associated diarrhea.

106. C: Intertrigo is most likely to occur in patients that are obese, especially in humid conditions. It results from the interaction of friction, moisture, and heat and often occurs in body folds with erythema, maceration, and fissures. Patients may experience pain, itching, and burning and may develop a secondary bacterial or fungal infection. The area must be kept clean and dry. Treatment includes topical steroids (hydrocortisone 1%) and an antifungal, such as clotrimazole 1%.

107. C: The most common cause of treatment-resistant acne vulgaris in adult females is polycystic ovary syndrome, which may also be characterized by hirsutism, virilism, and irregular menstrual periods. Typically, lesions vary and may include cysts, papules, and pustules most commonly located on the face, shoulders, upper back, upper chest, and neck. Some patients may develop extensive pitting and scarring over time.

108. A: With cellulitis, blood testing usually shows leukocytosis with increased neutrophils. Cellulitis is most common on the lower extremities but can occur elsewhere. Cellulitis typically initially appears as a small reddened edematous area that expands over the next 6–36 hours and is often accompanied by increasing fever and chills. In some cases, septicemia and hypotension may occur. Treatment is with IV or parenteral antibiotics. Cellulitis is usually caused by gram-positive cocci, such as group A beta-hemolytic streptococci, *Staphylococcus aureus,* and MRSA.

109. B: If, when conducting the history and physical exam of a new patient, the patient has multiple complaints and keeps interrupting the healthcare provider to discuss more issues, some major (abdominal pain) but some very minor (hangnail), the best response for the healthcare provider is to ask the patient to help prioritize problems. This may help the patient to focus on problems that are more severe, although problems that seem minor (such as fatigue) may be an indication of a serious health concern.

110. D: DIAPERS mnemonic:

D	Delirium	Acute delirium and the related confusion may cause acute urinary incontinence.
I	Infection	Especially urinary tract infection
A	Atrophic urethritis	May cause irritation and stress incontinence.
P	Pharmacy	Many drugs increase urinary retention and stress incontinence.
E	Excessive urine production	May be associated with disease, such as diabetes.
R	Restricted mobility	Inability to access toilet facilities
S	Stool impaction	May block flow of urine.

It's Your Moment, Let's Celebrate It!

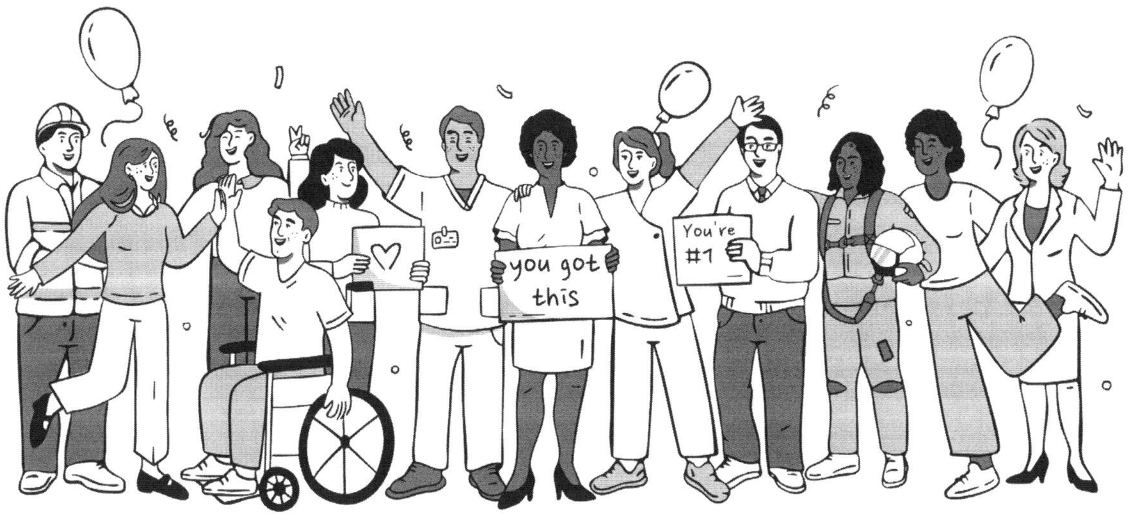

Share your story @mometrixtestpreparation